Pucker Power

Pucker Power

Great Kissers Make Great Lovers

Shelley Hess

Authors Choice Press

San Jose New York Lincoln Shanghai

Pucker Power
Great Kissers Make Great Lovers
All Rights Reserved © 2001 by Shelley Marleen Hess

Authors Choice Press
an imprint of iUniverse.com, Inc.

For information address:
iUniverse.com, Inc.
5220 S 16th, Ste. 200
Lincoln, NE 68512
www.iuniverse.com

ISBN: 0-595-17559-7

Printed in the United States of America

Dedication

I dedicate this book in memory of my "Guardian Angel", who was also my best friend and mother. Thanks for looking out for me.

My love to you always.

Contents

Part Two

Acknowledgements

This book could never have come to fruition without the help of several people. First and foremost are all the volunteers that shared with me their stories and opinions about romantic kissing. Second is my editor who offered support and guidance in getting all the kinks worked out. Last but not least are my sisters Jackie and Laurie who gave me the encouragement to finish the manuscript in the first place. To each and everyone of you my heart felt thanks.

Forward

I have known Shelley for a long time. She has always been a sensuous woman. From the first night we met, we enjoyed hours of great kissing.

She mentioned a kissing technique she learned when she was just nineteen that she uses to this very day. And even though she over analyzes everything, she was definitely right about knowing how to share a great sensuous kiss!

Sincerely,

Ted Hampton

Notes from the Author

The purpose of this book is entertainment and information. The stories told are based on "real-life" experiences. Since I am a single female over forty, I have a personal perspective on the art of kissing. I have had the opportunity to experience some incredible kisses as well as some incredibly awful ones too. As a holistic health practitioner, I have a wonderful clientele composed primarily of women. Many of them were kind enough to share with me their personal perspectives too. As I developed the manuscript, they were fascinated with the information. I hope you will find this enjoyable, informative and something to bring out the very best in your own personal kissing techniques.

The real identities have been changed to protect the privacy of those who were kind enough to share their lives with me.

In creating this book, I contacted many dentists and some orthodontists too. They were very helpful in supplying technical information about our mouths. When they learned why I was asking the questions, they offered their own personal opinions too. I want to express my thanks to each and every one of them, as well as to all the others who were so free with their own opinions and information. One thing I am certain is that kissing is a topic we all find interesting. I hope that you will take the material in this book and use it to bring more enjoyment into your personal lives. To each and every one of you my own personally written kiss. Remember GREAT kissing is the REAL "HOT SPOT" for great sex!

PART ONE

CHAPTER ONE

Finding Your Partner's "HOT SPOT"

The idea that men and women enter into a physical encounter with different agendas is not new or unexpected. It is a well-respected concept that men will approach sex on a physical level more often than women do. And women will approach sex on a more emotional level more often than men do. The frustration builds when the man and woman get together sexually and feel that their needs were not completely met.

Finding the "Hot Spot" to get both partners to feel that their needs were satisfied is the key to great sex. And that goal is where the art of kissing comes to the rescue. You do not have to worry about waiting for the "right place" to get each of you in the mood. Anywhere is perfect. So the fastest way to get men and women really turned on is with the first sensuous kiss.

Most of us begin practicing to kiss with the adolescent game called "spin-the-bottle". But none of us really know the way to kiss to make our first experiences really pleasurable. Sadly, some of us will spend all of our adult lives, never learning a good way to kiss.

Can you remember the first time you thought about wanting to be kissed? Did you worry if you would do it "right?" Most of us do. When we are young we do not have any previous experience. But the power behind our lips goes back to being a baby. Watch any infant and you will see that it will use its mouth as the center focus of its entire world. Babies place everything into their mouths, it is how they explore and learn. As adults our lips and tongue provide us with powerful sensations and reactions. A GREAT kiss is the BEST wonderful sensation of them all.

Being a single woman myself, I have gone on more "set-up dates" than I wish to confess. The desire to get a "wonderful" goodnight kiss was often not fulfilled. Then I began to ask all my female clients and friends about their experiences with kissing, and I soon realized that there are significant differences in the style and techniques used in kissing. Not to sound overly critical of men, but these women remember more "duds" than "fireworks" after being kissed. Hundreds of men did not have a clue that their expertise in kissing was leaving their partners "flat." How many times can you recall being pursued by a self-declared red-hot lover, and finding yourself looking for the door to make a quick escape? These are the same men that think that you will fall easily into their arms and off to bed. WRONG…sad to say that they do not have a clue as to what will make a sizzling kiss. There are some methods that can put you flying through the stratosphere. These are the ones I will share with you.

I want to draw your attention to the kind of kissing that will truly sexually stimulate both of you. Your primary consideration should be about kissing for the purpose of enjoying sex and sexual relationships.

Caressing and Kissing:

Humans are very tactile people. The next time you are in the shower, take a moment and run your fingertips over your arms, chest, stomach and torso. Notice how wonderful it feels. The desire to be touched goes way back to our very beginning of life. Expectant mothers can rub their bellies and the baby will calm down and enjoy this in-vitro massage. Did you know that you NEED some form of touch daily to be happy and well adjusted? Without caressing over a long period of time, you can become depressed and need medical help. It is a lot easier to just make sure you get at LEAST one good hug a day. It will be even more effective than "the old apple to keep the doctor away."

Caressing can be done by various methods using different parts of the body. Your fingers are the first part you use to give others that perfect caress. Your arms and upper torso are what is needed to give that wonderful "Bear Hug". Remember how safe and secure you felt inside your mother or father's arms when you were little?

But to feel romantic your caress begins with your mouth. Can you imagine using your own lips and tongue to create a wonderful caress?? If not, you don't know what you've been missing!! Your nerve endings on your tongue are highly sensitive and can be controlled to offer incredible sensations and reactions. Your lips can offer various amounts of pressure that can be very stimulating and arousing too.

During that perfect caress, you will use all four parts: fingers, arms, torso, and mouth. Can you picture how silly it would be to try to stimulate your partner without at least one embrace?

In a casual form of greeting hello or goodbye, it is common to offer a quick peck on the cheek or forehead without other body contact. This form of kissing is not generally described as an effective precursor to passion. The exception to this would be when a series of light pecks were made while the body contact intensified. Then the kissing changes to sexual kissing and the stimulation can begin.

The Sensual Kiss Is Worth More Than A Bushel & A Peck:

Up until a person reaches puberty, the only kind of kissing that s/he perform is the closed mouth kiss. The introduction of the use of the tongue during kissing is usually done in the pre-teen years. In the past, the average ten or eleven year old explores the art of Sensual Kissing in a clumsy and awkward fashion. Now in the 1990's, Sensual Kissing is shown on all soap dramas and evening sitcom programs. Any man, woman, or child can turn on their T.V. and get all the visual display in how a French Kiss is performed. You would think that people would now be able to perform the most exciting and stimulating kiss for their partners. Sad to say it simply is not true.

The following will seem to be anything but sensual in the way the Sensual Kiss is evaluated. Once you learn the actual technique, you will forget the mechanics of the kiss and relish it's power to arouse you and your partner.

Here are three key complaints about the typical kiss:

> First was the feeling that the person initiating the kiss just stuck their tongue in the other's mouth. Leaving it there as if it's presence was supposed to be exciting.
> Second was the excessive slobber that the receiving partner was forced to deal with during the kiss.
> Last was the total "turn-off" response the partner had while being kissed in this manner.

There is a genuine art to Sensual Kissing. The kiss is a form of exploration and a kind of dance between two peoples' mouths. The real connoisseur will work their lips and tongue in a method of exploring the other person's lips, teeth, gums, and tongue. The connoisseur will use his mouth as a tool. Although not terribly romantic, his mouth will work over his partner's carefully and slowly. He will take the time to touch every part of her mouth. The sensory capability of the mouth is huge. If properly manipulated, the nerve endings will send incredible waves of pleasure throughout your body.

You can use pressure with your lips along with the ability to playfully tug on your partner's lips to start the stimulation towards great sexual arousal. The introduction to seduction begins with the lips. Both partners are able to gauge the level of response from one another. Trouble arises when one or both forget to take the time to register the other's response. It is common for one partner to get caught up in their own reaction, forgetting to tune into their partner's response or lack of reaction. This person is so excited during the kiss that they fail to realize that the other person is not matching their enthusiasm. It may seem impossible for one of two people to be getting aroused with the kiss while the other has little or no reaction, but it happens a lot.

Egos get involved when kissing is done for sexual stimulation and arousal. The unaffected partner does not wish to complain to their partner about the "lousy kissing", for fear of hurting their feelings. The pattern of bad kissing simply continues on and on and on. Some people do not know how to offer a critique that will not shatter the other's ego. Some bad kissers simply do not have a clue how to improve. Their partners may not know how to guide them to do a better job. This book will be their guide.

Most of us begin practicing to kiss with the adolescent game called "spin-the-bottle". But none of us really know the way to kiss to make our first experiences really pleasurable. Sadly, some of us will spend all of our adult lives, never learning a good way to kiss….Here is an example of the power of not knowing how to execute a kiss, this is a re-telling of an actual event:

Leo was tall for his age, so his twelve and thirteen year old buddies never knew that he had just turned ten last weekend. He was excited about attending Tommy's party. It would be his first Girl-Boy party. He was not sure what made this different from the other parties he had gone too. Other girls in his class had gone to the other parties. When Tommy turned the lights off in the basement, and everyone sat in a circle, Leo sensed that something was different. He sat along side of his five pals while six girls sat giggling across the way. An empty coke bottle laid in the center of the ring. Spin-the-Bottle was a game he had never heard of before. He prayed he wouldn't have to take a turn going into the laundry room. But his prayers were not answered and Brita was his lucky selection. She was the tallest girl in the room and had very large breasts. It was nearly impossible to keep from staring at her chest. All the guys were hooting while they slowly made it to the laundry door. Leo wanted something to happen to put an end to this game. He didn't care what, just anything….Once they were inside the laundry room, Brita stuck her tongue in his mouth. He wanted to throw up. Brita ran out of the room, laughing and screaming "Leo doesn't even know how to French". Everyone else began to laugh, while Leo ran out of the house. He spent the rest of the evening at the curb, until his dad came to pick him up. It wasn't until he turned twelve, that Leo finally understood the game called spin-the-bottle. Being an only child, Leo didn't have anyone to ask these questions. It wasn't until he was in high school that Leo learned about French kissing. His childhood memories kept him from really liking it much. Leo never learned how to perform a good French Kiss.

Tips And Tricks For A Zinger Of A Kiss:

Start the Sensual Kiss with a playful tug on the bottom lip. This begins your journey towards a wonderful experience. The general rule of thumb is to begin with light pressure and tugging. (Different levels of pressure and pulling will be received as positive or negative.) In small increments, increase the force of your pressure or pulling on the bottom lip. Check your partner's reaction, do they seem to be enjoying it?

If they are, then the next step is sucking on their lip. Take your partner's bottom lip into your mouth and suckle it. This creates a lot of wonderful sensations. Your partner now realizes that you are full of surprises, and quite playful too. Although you might be thinking this all seems a bit unusual, it starts the kiss going in a suggestive manner. (A small note of caution: Your partner has to know that you will not bite down on their lip to cause them pain.) The sense of trust can be very exciting.

Follow the suckling of the bottom lip with the use of your tongue around their bottom gum line.* You do not need to be in a dentist chair to know how many nerve endings are in the gums. The soft tissue inside of the mouth is filled with incredibly powerful nerve relays. Exploring them with your tongue will make your partner come alive.

SOME KEY POINTS TO KEEP IN MIND:

When working your tongue inside of your partner's mouth, it is VERY IMPORTANT to keep control of your tongue.

Stuffing your tongue into your partner's mouth can be disenchanting to them.

The proper way to conduct your movement is with the tip of your tongue. Extending your tongue past your teeth will automatically force your tongue to be firmer. This will increase the control of movement you have with your tongue.

Pay CLOSE ATTENTION to the amount of saliva that will build up in both of your mouths. BE COURTEOUS and allow time to swallow. Drowning in drool, is one of the most common mistakes poor kissers make. (Refer to Chapter Eight)

*The following is not effective with full dentures. If either partner wears dentures, this technique will not have a positive reaction. The nerve endings are not exposed with a full denture pallet. The concern for slippage of the denture pallet will make either partner feel uneasy.

With your tongue extended, slide the tip of your tongue along the front side of your partner's lower teeth. In order to NOT create a "tickling sensation," apply direct, firm pressure. This movement will make your partner relax their jaw and be enticed to allow further exploration of your tongue.

The next movement will be to take the tip of your tongue and glide it behind the front teeth and under your partner's tongue. The normal reaction is to have the receiver move their tongue forward. As this happens guide their tongue past their teeth to move into your mouth. Press your lips around your partner's tongue and apply a sucking pressure against their tongue to gain further control over your partner's tongue. Suckle their tongue for several minutes. Make sure you pay attention to the amount of saliva that builds up under the tongue. By placing the top of your tongue under the bottom of your partner's tongue, you can return their tongue to their mouth without breaking contact.

With your tongue back in your partner's mouth, run the tip of your tongue on the upper pallet. This area can be very **TICKLISH**, so make your pressure **very firm**.

Next move around your partner's top teeth and gum line. You can use both sides of your tongue while doing this part of the kiss.

This style of kissing awakens the nerve endings in your partner's mouth, tongue and lips. Your partner is made aware of how detailed your technique is to arousing their body. Here are just a few of the messages your technique is offering:

I don't want to rush our time together.
I enjoy giving your body time to react to me.
I enjoy caressing you.
More is yet to come…. This makes your partner want to share with you, too. You have set the stage for a great love making session. An even more terrific, pleasurable experience awaits for both of you to enjoy.

Here is an example of the power of the mouth, this is a re-telling of another actual event:

Zoe was sitting at her usual table. She found herself coming to Boddy's Bar every Friday for happy hour the last two years. The crowd was like an extended family of sorts. Most of the regulars knew a lot about her. Maybe she should have been more closed-lipped. But then again, lips were her passion. Everything about the mouth interested, Zoe. In turn, she often found herself running-off-at-the-mouth, so to speak. She loved the way her tongue moved around her mouth and lips, as she spoke. Not too many people thought that lips were the most sexual feature on the body. Zoe felt that breasts, legs, and butts were largely over-rated, while the uniqueness of most peoples' mouths went unnoticed. Lips were her favorite part of anyone's body. Zoe thought of herself as a "people-watcher" of their mouths. Tonight was not any different. The room was filled with gray smoke. That did not stop Zoe from noticing the stranger that was seated at the bar. He seemed oblivious to the crowd, as he worked the exhaled cigarette smoke into precise rings. To do so, he was extending his bottom lip into the air. It was driving Zoe crazy. Zoe watched his mouth with the same intensity, as he did on the smoke rings. Zoe could feel her heartbeat beginning to quicken. **This** Friday night might end up interesting after all......... Now Zoe had to find a way to get his attention. He already had hers. She wasn't a smoker, so she couldn't just walk over to his table and ask for a cigarette. Zoe looked around to see if anyone else in the bar seemed to recognize this erotic stranger. Perhaps she could then ask them to provide her with an introduction. Unfortunately no one seemed to be even a bit interested in looking over in his direction. The more she watched him and the actions of his lips on the cigarette, the more excited she was getting. What seemed like an hour was in fact only seven minutes. Zoe was beside herself, she just had to make contact with this man. Her desire to feel his lips on hers was growing by the seconds that passed. In desperation, she just walked over to his table and said: "I have been watching how skillfully you make smoke rings with your cigarette. Would you mind if I watched you from here?". John looked at her with surprise in his eyes and a genuine smile on his lips. (He did not introduce himself, so she didn't know his name at this moment.) He was pleased to have her notice him.

As Zoe and John retold their first meeting to me, they both agreed to the above details. Then each had their own version of what happened after she sat next to him.

ZOE: She remembers sitting there for an incredibly long time just watching him blow smoke rings. He didn't appear to be interested in talking much less letting her play with his lips. Sitting so close and not being able to touch his mouth with hers was driving her mad. She waited until he had finished his cigarette, and as he was reaching for another, she reached over and kissed him directly on the mouth. Not knowing what his reaction was going to be, she couldn't just begin her approach with her suckling his lips. That would be her next move, if given the opportunity. She was thrilled that John didn't pull away. Zoe and John sat kissing and kissing for the remainder of the time Boddy's was open. She was so turned on, she thought she would jump out of her skin. Zoe asked him over to her place, and was thrilled that he seemed eager to go.

John: He remembers sitting in the bar for a matter of moments, before Zoe came over to where he was sitted. He was shocked and pleased at the very same time. She was attractive and attentive to detail. Having her sit and watch him didn't bother him a bit. Just as he was getting into setting up a series of rings, something he got a kick out of doing, she jumped over to him and kissed him. Now this really surprised him, but he definitely did NOT mind a bit! John remembers necking like school kids until the bar closed. The kissing was very passionate and when she invited over to her place, he was ready to go....

The anticipation of a great kiss is very erotic. You do not have to have a fetish about lips at all. On a scale, a great kiss is worth more than its weight in solid gold. The right kiss will lead into a wonderful physical encounter. It does not have to be actual intercourse, although it certainly could move to making love. Since men relate to sex with less emotions than most women do, the act of kissing levels out the imbalance. It is easy to relate kissing on any level. Both partners can enjoy it on a physical level with or without the emotions. Then if the emotions do get charged up, the kissing can flow with the feelings just as easily.

Sensual Kissing can be such a glorious kind of kiss. The variety alone can offer hours of enjoyment. Here is how it started for another couple I spoke with:

> There was a full moon shining as Ted and Alice walked from the campus library back to their dorms. They had spent several hours pouring over their books. Each kept stealing glimpses of the other while in the library. Ted was wondering how it would be to lay naked over Alice's body, while Alice was dreaming of being held tightly in Ted's arms. Both were having their own sexual fantasies, which lead to the French Kissing outside on the dorm's porch. After twenty minutes of kissing, Alice floated upstairs to her room, while Ted went in to take a very cold shower.

CHAPTER TWO

Lips

The size and shape of your lips can be a major attraction for your partner. From the inquiries I made, it was suggested that lips with more fullness were considered to be sexy.

> Having "pout-y" lips seemed to indicate the person would be considered sexier than others without "pout-y" looking mouths. Another style of lips that were considered most sexy were lips that had the lower lip being full while the upper lip was thinner. The lips that were rated to be the least sexy were thin on the top and bottom and the entire mouth was small in size.

Lip shapes come in as many varieties as there are people. Heredity plays a large role into the reasons why this is so. However, two parents can have several children and each will have their own unique lip characteristics. Not as unique as our fingerprints, they still have elements that make them special. These multiple varieties differ in size as well as in their shape. Some people have very full lips, while others have very thin ones. Lips can be balanced top and bottom or may appear mis-matched. A lot of people will have a fuller bottom lip than the top one. Make up artists will use cosmetics to help women appear to have more symmetry to their mouths. A few people may argue that fuller lips offer a more sensuous feeling while kissing. However, thin lips can create a wonderful kissing sensation too. Some people may simply have a preference to the size and shape of their partner's mouth. Remember that the actual shape of our lips rarely limits our kissing abilities. Anyone can be a great kisser.

Mysteries of Your Mouth Revealed:

Ever wonder makes your mouth so flexible? It is able to move in so many different shapes due to a muscle with a funny name: the Obicularis Oris. It is a curricular muscle with several bands that run on the top of the lip and on the bottom. It does wear out easily and shows the aging process sooner than most of us would desire. Plastic surgery is not an option because of the circular formation. The usual cutting and tightening methods do not work. But if you are worried about your mouth looking less youthful, here is a list of solutions you can use:

> Laser treatments work to renew a youthful appearance of the mouth.
> Dermabrasion, or Chemical peels performed with phenol acid, Jessner's solution, and/or glycolic acids make the aging skin around the lips more attractive.

These treatments are being performed on men and women, by dermatologists, plastic surgeons, and some clinically trained estheticians.

There are some that believe that an exercise program called ISOMETRICS can improve the strength of the muscle. I have found no evidence to prove this claim. IF isometrics is supposed to create a stronger muscle tone by working on the muscles of the mouth, then smokers should have very firm mouth tissue. BUT they do not!

Besides heredity, smoking and exposure to the sun are the two most damaging elements to make your mouth appear less youthful. Although the reduction of tone of your mouth is not eye-appealing, it does not effect the ability to be a great kisser.

Sensuous FULL Lips:

Several years ago in France, it was discovered that a woman could go and have her lips increased in size with the help of a doctor. The idea caught on through the publicity in fashion magazines. The "FRENCH LIPS" became the rage. With the use of injectable collagen, anyone can now have fuller lips. This procedure is only performed by a doctor, and it is only temporary. The body will absorb the collagen, and the process must be repeated two times a year to maintain the appearance of full lips.

The size of the lips can play a minor role in the effectiveness of a kiss. The technique of what is done with the lips rather than the size of the lips was more important. The texture of the lips did have a very significant impact on the effects of the kisses. Smooth, soft lips provide a better reaction than rough, chapped lips. I believe that using products to keep the lips healthy is a wise investment.

A special story about the uniqueness of the lips comes from Sondra and Mack. Theirs was completely different than Zoe and John:

> To most people their meeting was an ironic twist of fate, but to Mack meeting Sondra was kismet (fate/ meant-to-be). Sondra was a volunteer book reader for the Braille Institute, and Mack worked as the custodian. For four years, Sondra would record for the books-on-tape program from her house. Then one evening her house was robbed and she no longer had a tape recorder. Because of her heavy work schedule, Sondra couldn't make it to the Institute to do the recording there. So she

dropped out of the program for one year. In that time, Mack began to want to go back and get his degree. He also had a tough time making the time to study. Mack made an arrangement with the Braille Institute to be able to use the tapes to study, while no one else was using them. Mack was the in-house custodian of the Institute. He would play them as he did his cleaning late at night. Mack had never met Sondra, but he fell in love with her through her tapes. Her voice melted into his brain and heart. Although he had never actually seen Sondra, he was certain he would recognize her by her mouth. While listening to her voice every single night for one year, he had a picture of what her lips and mouth would look like. He fantasized about what it would be like to kiss her. He dreamt about her each and every night. Then one evening he heard his fantasy lady's voice coming out of one of the recording rooms. At first he dismissed it as just one of the students listening to one of the many pre-recorded tapes. But suddenly she stopped, another voice was speaking. His fantasy lady was actually here in person!!! Someone was talking to her! He could barely believe it, and yet he found himself glued to the spot he was standing. He became frightened to actually be able to see her face-to-face. Filled with total self-doubt, he couldn't bring himself to go and meet her. He did not even know her name. Suddenly, he heard someone call out "Sondra". It became the most beautiful name he had ever heard. For two weeks he pondered what he would be able to do, if given the opportunity to meet her again. Mack was given the chance, but not by his own doing. The administrator of the school called him into the office to fix an electrical socket, when Sondra was already in the room. He was introduced to her, and all he could do was nod his head and stare at her lips. They were as perfect as he had imagined. She had a full bottom lip and a smooth gentle curve on her top lip. She wasn't wearing any lipstick but they were an incredible light pink color. He was starring so hard that Sondra and his boss asked if something was wrong? How could Mack explain the circumstances that had caused his behavior? He simply stammered and left the room. He felt so ridiculous and wanted to kick himself, so he took out his frustrations on the lockers near by. Sondra heard the commotion and went out to find out if one of the students were in trouble. Finding Mack in such a state, she decided to ask if everything was alright or if she could help? That began their life-long romance. Sondra retells how Mack will take her in his arms and kiss her for hours. She had never had anyone take such pleasure in exploring her lips and mouth. The power of the lips can last forever.

Soft, Smooth Lips:

From a woman's point of view, the condition of the lips had a direct effect on the success of the kiss. If you suffer from cracked dry lips, you can do more than just living with the condition. Here are several ways to make your lips soft and smooth. It begins with replacing the water that your lips need to stay moist.

Did you know that you NEED those eight glasses of water on a daily basis to stay healthy? There is not a single part of your body that does not need water, even your bones do. If the idea of swallowing that much water seems too large a task to do, try to start slowly with the following program.

Drink one glass of water for two days
Drink two glasses of water for two days
Drink three glasses of water for three days
Drink four glasses of water for four days

Drink five glasses for five days—by this time your body will be desiring the water and it won't be such a task.
Drink six glasses for six days
Drink seven glasses for seven days
Drink eight glasses for eight days

You can add slices of lemon, lime or orange rinds to the water to make it taste better. Using bottled or filtered water will also help. Putting your water in a gorgeous cut crystal glass will bring your attention to drinking it.

Licking your lips will also cause the skin to peel. There are skin care techniques to remove the cracked peeled skin off of your lips. Professional cosmetic companies have created lip exfoliators that will remove the dead, flaky skin. The skin underneath will be soft and smooth. Coating your lips with waxy cover sticks are not a good solution. They make the surface feel smooth but actually the wax cuts off the oxygen from the lip surface which will cause the skin to continue to crack and peel.

Read Her Lips:

For all the men that have had trouble understanding the specific elements of their partner's personality, this guide will be especially helpful. Crazy as it will may appear, it WORKS. Forget calling your psychic hotline, to get advice how to deal with the women in your life….sneak into their makeup bags and get out their lipstick tubes. Check the shape of the lipstick to the following designs and follow this guide…

I collected my information during a psychology course in college. I had all the females on campus participate, over 2,000 in all. I published the results in my thesis for the class. Since then I have used this information when dealing with my clients. It has been accurate 98% of the time.

1. ORIGINAL SLANT—A bit reserved and self-conscious, she will follow the leader rather than be the leader herself. She's loyal and will want to be in a long-term relationship. She will accept a casual relationship only in the beginning. Once it gets romantic, the commitment has been made.

2. ROUNDED ETCHED POINT—Rather nit-picky and precise. She is very family-oriented, placing them above all else. She loves to be surrounded by loved ones and friends. Treat her well and she will be faithful in hard times and easy ones.

3. CREW CUT—She always runs on schedule and has little patience when things do not flow on time. Her standards and morals are high and she is decisive. Ironically, however she will look towards her partner for approval about her appearance. Once you earn her trust, she will be loyal, but you will really have to prove yourself worthy.

4. SMOOTH AND ROUND—The moment you met her, you probably felt like you had known her all of your life. Every one of her friends feels this way. She's easy to talk too. Never balks if you're running late and will go the extra-mile to keep the peace. She is generous with her time and her belongings. Sometimes you may wish she wasn't so willing to share herself with those around you. She has a hard time telling her close friends and family not to come around. Even when you might want it to be just the "two-of-you".

5. JAGGED EDGE—She's lively, creative, talkative and spontaneous. She'll put you behind schedule or leave you waiting for her to get ready. However, she is do full of life and her bubbly personality, usually wins you over. At a party, she is often the center of attention, due to her strong speaking skills. Conversations with her are long but never boring.

6. THE PEAK—She will be highly spiritual and her faith is very important. Accepting her strong beliefs will gain you a committed and faithful partner. She will expect you to be faithful as well. In fact she will accept nothing less. She is passionate about her family, children, and will be especially about her husband (when/if she marries). Although she enjoys the lime-light, she always seeks approval from her partner. IF you make her feel like a queen, she will do ANYTHING to make you feel like a king.

7. CREW CUT WITH A DIP—She is so full of curiosity, that she asks endless amounts of questions about everything. This can get to be very annoying over time. If you make the time to offer her answers to the big questions, she will let the smaller issues slide. She will be happy to read up on any topic that you find interesting to learn more about it. To get her to stop interrupting your favorite sporting event, with questions to what is going on and why, send her to the library to read up on the sport before you take her to a game, or watch it on TV.

8. CLIFFHANGER-She has an opinion on everything and she's always right. Or so she sees it that way. She makes up her mind very slowly, so give her time to do so. Or do not give her too many choices to decide on. She likes attention from others, and sometimes gets in trouble because her friendliness is interrupted as flirting. She does not see her behavior as anything but being sociable. Often it is a challenge to please her because she takes so long to make up her mind what she likes and does not like. She tends to change her opinions a lot, and sometimes in different directions from the first position she held.

Do not be alarmed if your partner has several different tubes of lipstick and they might have DIFFERENT SHAPES. People respond differently to colors. How she feels when she is wearing red can be quite different when she is wearing chocolate brown or peach. Since most of us have several different components that make up our personalities, learning all of them takes time. Take note of each tube's distinctive shape and watch how she acts when wearing each shade of lipstick. You can then gauge how to deal with her depending on her reactions. IF one behavior is more pleasing to you than others, you can then subtly suggest that she wear the color you like her behavior to best.

CHAPTER THREE

The Sense of Touch

WHAT IS "GOOD TOUCH"?

In the attempt to avoid the wrong contact, we have removed from our daily routine what is called the "GOOD TOUCH". It is what we all can do for each other. It can offer a person a feeling of sexuality, or it can fill the need to express caring and thoughtful expression through the ability to kiss, hug, caress or hold someone.

There has been a lot of publicity about "BAD TOUCHING" which involves the problems associated with pedifiles, and other deviants. Unfortunately, to keep our children safe from harms way, our society has become closed to the idea of open touching of one another. For many reasons this ideology has proven to be necessary and has a great deal of merit.

The need to be cared for and shown affection begins in infancy. Many magazines like **Parenting, and Ladies Home Journal** report studies done with infants that are raised with only their biological needs fulfilled. They are fed, bathed, clothed and provided shelter. They are not given any form of personal interaction, or affection shown to them in any way. The babies grow up with behavioral problems, and are not well adjusted children.

In a lot of households throughout the nation, we will find single—parent relationships that do not have the convenience to get a warm hug "hello" from a mate. If you were to check with neighbors and family associates, you would be told how busy everyone is, and therefore no one has the time to seek out a daily kiss or embrace from a friend, significant other, or relative.

Adolescents in this generation, do not think it's "cool" to come home and kiss and/or hug their parent(s). They are too busy to go to their rooms for their own private space, and private communication amongst their own peers. In fact children over the age of nine, will probably not make time to kiss or hug their parent(s) goodnight.

The average person will have other normal stresses in their lives that keep them too busy to seek out daily caresses. Kisses and hugs are one of the best use of touch, for your own health and well-being. Beginning with a warm embrace, followed with a kiss is the perfect remedy for a stressful day.

The kiss can begin the process of "good touching". Your partner gets the feedback that you care about them. From that moment on, your relationship begins to build with each other. It is never too soon to create the bond that will make the relationship last.

As we age, the need for hugs does not go away, it only increases. The ability to fulfill the need gets harder.

Several years ago, there was an ad campaign created through the United States Health and Welfare department. Bumper stickers and billboards were created with the phrase: "Have You Hugged Your Child Today?". It was so well received that mock stickers were created with phrases of all

kinds, Have you hugged your teddy bear today?, Have you hugged your
_____ today?(every breed of dog and cat was placed in this question/
sentence.)

A whole organization called "The Touch For Health" was started that
promoted "group hugs". They felt that everyone should go around asking total strangers if they need a hug. They made up T-shirts that had a
symbol of two hands grasping each other on one side, and two people
hugging on the other, with the question "Do you need a hug?". They
were open to the idea that anyone could approach them for a hug.

Some people felt that it was part of the "Love Child" movement of the
sixties. No matter where or why they were started, it made people aware
of the need to have someone show that they cared. Seminars were created by the group, where the attendees could spend a whole weekend at
a retreat. While they were away with the group, they got their fill of
attention. In the real world of their daily lives, it was not so easy to find
a resource for such attention.

Ask yourself these questions:

> Is there hesitation in the way you allow your lips to touch
> someone?
> Do you offer a hug timidly?

Answering YES to these questions means you might need to work on
making your partner feel secure around you.

> Do you try to offer just your finger tips, when someone else
> offers an outstretched palm?
> Do you provide a "wet noodle" kind of handshake?

These are signs that you are not ready to have someone get too personal.

Check to see if this is how your partner responds. It is possible that they are not ready to have you get too close. You need to be sensitive to their reactions.

It may NOT be a direct response to you. You have to remember that your partner may have events in their past that make reaching out to you difficult. Previously in their lives, it might have been impossible to express warm feelings. So greet them with a warm smile, firm embrace and a great kiss.

The ability to get so close is just one more reason that the "good touching" is a vital element to creating the bond and trust between you and your lover.

When you go to extend your hands on their bodies, it is important to have your fingers and nails look clean, healthy, and smooth. Remember that your hands are a direct reflection of you to your lover. Who would want to be touched by a lobster claw? Or worse yet, a dirty, smelly, lobster claw? IF you smoke, remember that the tar and nicotine resins will stay on your hands. Make sure that you keep a nail brush handy to scrub under your nails several times throughout the day.

CHAPTER FOUR

Searching for the Great Lover

A. Looking at Yourself

Most every woman will have difficulty looking at themselves naked in a mirror and liking what they see. Typically a person will able to offer negative reactions to the image in the mirror. Women are quicker to offer negative feedback about their naked bodies than men. With my volunteers, everyone had some comment about their features that they would want to see changed. Over 72% listed "faults" in their appearances. 100% listed the negative reactions first. It was only during my one-on-one consultation with each of them, did they then add their positive reactions.

The trend was to look for the "negative" when gazing into a mirror, rather than seeking out the "positive". This has a direct effect on how you will interact with your own 'significant other'. Men and women are more likely to criticize ones' appearance than to praise it. Each physical characteristic was picked apart. Noses were the feature that had the most negative comments. Tied for the second most disliked feature were eyebrows and chins, then came lips, cheeks, and the one feature that had the least negative comments on were the eyes. In fact the most favored feature on everyone's face was their eyes. This follows the old Chinese proverb "The Eyes Are The Windows To The Soul". All in all, people are very critical of themselves. Based on my volunteers, it can be said that you will be much more generous when judging another person's physical appearance than you will of your own. The expression "To Thy Own Self Be True, might be better changed to read "To Thy Own Self Be KIND"!

When a man and woman get together for the first time, their negative reactions about themselves effects their interaction together. If one or both have too strong a negative opinion about their own appeal, they will not easily engage in intimate contact. Kissing is considered an intimate contact.

To enjoy kissing, you have to be comfortable with yourself. This does not mean that you have to want to kiss your own reflection every time you pass a mirror. You do have to make it a priority to work on your own self confidence. It is important to accent the positives not the negatives.

When we watch a TV program and see all the actors and actresses with pearl-white, perfectly shaped teeth, we can't help but notice how beautiful their mouths look. The likelihood that all of them were blessed with perfect natural teeth is close to impossible. In reality, they spent thousands of dollars on cosmetic dentistry to obtain their appearance of a flawless mouth. However a perfect set of teeth does not always make for a fantastic smile. The feeling behind the smile can have more to do with the way the other person reacts than the cosmetic presentation.

You have probably met a man or woman that had such a "warm smile" that their whole face "lit up" while they were smiling. This person can

have very crooked teeth, or ones that are not pearly-white in color.
Regardless, when we are in their company and they smile at us, we
know that they are genuinely interested in us. We can feel the warmth
and good feelings through their expressions. This person is going to
make us feel comfortable enough to want to get close and kiss, and
kiss, and kiss some more. Their genuine charm effects our reactions.
This is the goal all of us must meet to make our partners feel comfortable to be close and personal. It is more important to feel fondness
than it is to look perfect.

The old cliché: "A picture is worth a thousand words", has a direct sig-
nificance in relating to kissing. A great kissing embrace can start with
wonderful eye contact first. If there is a twinkle in the eye, it will say so
much more to our partners than perfect words. Not everyone is comfortable with verbal expressions of affection. Some people find it easier
to use body contact to express themselves. Kissing becomes an easy way
to say the words that do not come out comfortably. If you have a tough
time saying the words "I love you", you can express your affection with a
kiss. Great kissing does make for great romance. Here is a re-telling how
it created a wonderful romance for Lorraine and Alfred. Theirs is a tale
that just proves how Pucker Power can change one's life….

Lorraine walked to the same outdoor cafe everyday during
work, for lunch. She loved to get some fresh air and watch the
people as she eat her home-made sandwich. All of sudden
she noticed a man watching her watch everyone else. She
began to feel self-conscious. Did she make others feel this
way?. It had never occurred to her before. As she was deep in
self-contemplation, the man walked over to her table and
asked to sit down. Lorraine's first reaction was to refuse him,
but he flashed her a smile that would have melted an iceberg.
She couldn't help herself from reacting to it's warmth and
nodded a yes. As he sat down, he extended his hand and said,

"My name is Alfred, and I noticed that you are a people watcher too". As he took Lorraine's hand, he gave her another "hot" smile.

They preceded to chat through her entire lunch break. The hour sped by so quickly, she couldn't believe she had to go back to work. Not wanting to appear too forward she debated whether to offer her phone number. It wasn't to be a problem, because Alfred reached into his briefcase and pulled out an organizer. He asked for her business card. When she did not have one, he asked for her number so that he could log it in. She gave him her office number, since he hadn't actually asked for her home number. Then she decided she really did have to get back to work, so she stood up. And as she did, Alfred reached over and kissed her on the cheek, close to her ear actually. His lips were as warm as his smile had been. She could still feel his lips on her skin, and it made her feel warm inside. Lorraine couldn't wait to hear or see him again. His kiss provoked a feeling of excitement she had not experienced in a long time. She walked back to her office with her mind reeling. Lorraine filled her thoughts with visions of kissing Alfred the next day at lunch-time. Would it happen? Could it happen?...By the end of the work day, she was looking forward to the next lunch break more than she had ever wanted another day of work to come. Usually she was always looking forward to the work day to end, and dreading how quickly the next work schedule always would come along. Alfred's kiss had changed all that.

Lorraine rushed down to the cafe, hoping that she could find Alfred. In just a few moments she saw that he was indeed sitting in the plaza. When their eyes met, he offered his melting smile and Lorraine felt her knees begin to grow weak. Now would not be the time to fall down. Alfred met her in the middle of the court yard and immediately put his hand under her elbow. It was as if he could sense the reaction his smile was having on her. As he leaned towards her to plant another kiss on her temple, Lorraine turned her head to meet his lips with her own. She wasn't planning to be so aggressive with her actions. But she did not regret the decision as soon as she felt his lips on hers. Alfred was a great kisser. He moved his mouth over hers as if he owned hers. The pressure he asserted was not too strong or too weak. He was the perfect kisser, and she couldn't bring herself to break away, and kissing in public wasn't something she did a lot. In fact her co-workers could be staring at her blatant display of affection. Regardless, it didn't stop her, she was enjoying the kiss that much. When they finally broke away, neither knew exactly what to say. They decided to grab a slice of pizza and take a stroll down the street. That began a relationship that is still going strong.

Sometimes you have to take chances and do things that you might not otherwise consider doing to make changes in your life. Clearly Lorraine and Alfred did not expect to meet each other, nor did either of them know that they would be able to relate to each other with the innocent kiss on the temple. But kissing can be a very powerful force, and great kissing is incredible. It does take two to make it work well. Which leads to the other part of the evaluation process, the other partner....

B. Looking at your partner

For whatever reasons, we tend to be less critical of our mates. They can have weak chins, crooked teeth, or thin lips and it doesn't seem to be as big a deal than if we have the same characteristics. However bad breath is one element that is NOT acceptable for either partner. (Refer to Chapter Eight.)

If your partner is able to get you to respond to their way of kissing, then you are on your way to a very healthy and happy physical relationship. The real trouble lays in the area of having to tell your partner that their technique in kissing is leaving you flat, high and dry, or feeling out on a limb. No matter how you say it, it just seems to be a hard thing to express. Ego is part of the reason. We are all very fragile when it comes to our egos and being told that your kissing style is not good certainly does not help establish a feeling of peace and harmony.

Most of us have never taken a course in the proper way to kiss. You can take lessons to learn how to be a better business person, how to cook, how to listen more effectively, how to talk in public, how to dance, how to sing, how to speak another language, how to read body language, how to give a sensuous massage, but I have never found a course in how to be a better KISSER. And I searched many data bases to find any course on the subject and found NONE. It is my opinion that a course would be very helpful to a lot of people. It is the reason for this book.

Kissing can be a wonderful way to communicate to another person. Your partner can learn so much about you through kissing you. But how do you tell your partner that you do not enjoy their kissing technique?.... It would be difficult for most of us to just come out and say "I do not like the way you kiss?". I was in fact in this exact predicament. I was in a wonderful relationship with a man who's kissing style was anything but pleasant. Not knowing how to properly handle the situation, I tried to bring up the subject asking if he had ever tried other ways to kiss? His immediate reaction was to tell me that he didn't get any complaints from other women, and preceded to stop kissing me all together for six months. I tried on numerous occasions to break the "boycott" by initiating a kiss. But this man only pulled away and stopped my advances. Ironically the relationship did not end, it lasted for over twelve years. But a twelve year relationship without great kissing can not be as fulfilling as a shorter one that includes it.

In hindsight, I should NOT have asked a direct question at all. I should have chosen a time when we were both in a very intimate situation and initiated a kiss in a style that I liked. When both partners are in the middle of a sexual experience, they are more receptive to trying new approaches and techniques with each other. Had this been done, I would not have bruised his ego. When it comes to a man's ego, they are definitely the "weaker sex"! This can be a costly lesson, take it from me, it is definitely worth walking on eggs, before preceding with total honesty. Which brings up another question, what if your partner asks you to tell them if you enjoy how they kissed you? Do you answer their inquiry with a NO? Absolutely NOT!!! Instead I recommend that you answer that you like many different kissing styles, theirs being one of them. And then offer to share with your partner the other ways you like to kiss. If they are receptive enough to want to get your feedback, they will be receptive enough to learn the new ways you kiss them.

CHAPTER FIVE

How to Become a Superb Kisser

The keys to unlocking a great kiss.

From all of my interviewing here are several specific points that were brought up a lot. Here they are in order of their importance.

1) Enjoy Kissing
2) Being Spontaneous
3) Physical Affection
4) Fresh Breath
5) Smooth Lips
6) Tongue Power
7) Dry Kisses
8) Exciting Pressure
9) Letting Up For Air
10) Unleashing The Fire In Your Partner's Body

Enjoy Kissing: You do not have to put it in words. You just feel it. It is a sense that is very powerful. Remember that BOTH of you have to really want to kiss.

Remember the author's personal friend and his reaction to her asking about changing their kissing style.

Being Spontaneous: You can plan your techniques to execute a kissing style. But when you actually engage in the actual kissing, it should come naturally and without it being a staged event.

Express Affection: Both of you need to be comfortable with expressing affection and feelings of love through body contact. Kissing and hugging are the two forms of physical contact that are the first ways to let each other know that you care a lot for each other.

Fresh Breath: The cliché "Fresh breath is kissing sweet" really says it all. Every one wants to have fresh breath when they are close to other people. Certainly kissing brings anyone close. Therefore a great kisser will always make sure that they have fresh breath before they begin to kiss.

Here is the retelling of one of the participants that was always concerned about how their breath smelled.

> Cleo was always worrying about her breath. She felt that her breath was always stale. Although she never sought out medical care to determine if she had a condition called "halitosis". Instead she decided to take care of her breath by eating lemon flavored hard candy. Cleo kept lemon drops in her purse, desk drawer, and even her glove box in her car. She never went anywhere without them. Although she wasn't aware of it, keeping the acidic candy in her mouth all day and most of the evening, contributed to the decay of all of her teeth. Cleo was constantly having to have her teeth drilled by her dentist. Fresh breath is a necessary component for a great kiss, but Cleo was so overly concerned about her lack of fresh breath, that she destroyed her own teeth.

Parsley would be a safer choice for keeping your breath fresh while protecting your teeth from acidic decay. It comes in tablet form and in it's natural raw form, it can be chewed and swallowed.

Smooth Lips: The skin on the lips are twice as thick as the skin on the rest of the face. The lips do not have any oil glands as the rest of the face does. A lot of people lick their lips often. Doing so will make them crack. Your own saliva will dry your lips out. When you spend a lot of time kissing, the exchange of saliva will also make your lips crack and dry. Kissing a soft, smooth surface is certainly more desirable than dry, cracked or peeling surface. Conditioning your lips will definitely pay off in a big way, particularly when wanting to be a great kisser.

Tongue Power: Most people do not realize how much variety there is to the shape of peoples' tongues along with the level of flexibility. Some have more flexible tongues than others. I always remember seeing my uncle fold his tongue in both directions. I tried and tried and could never do it at all. Anyone that speaks Spanish can roll their tongues too. My tongue was just not that flexible. However, everyone has the ability to control the movement of their tongues.

When you want to be an accomplished kisser, control is important. You need to use the tip of your tongue to work over your partner's mouth, tongue, teeth, and gums. If you keep your tongue flabby, it feels awful in your partner's mouth. This is what a lot of people forget!! You have to keep your attention on what your tongue feels like to your partner. By extending your tongue forward, allows the muscle to tighten. Lifting your tongue up past your teeth, rather than letting your teeth support the weight of your tongue, will also allow the muscle to tighten.

Having a toned, tightened body is more desirable than a flabby one. You have to keep your tongue tight and firm. Kissing is most enjoyable when both of you are in control....

Dry Kisses: It is inevitable to share our saliva with your partner during a passionate kiss. And you have to remember that your bacteria may not be as compatible with your partner's body as it is with your own. Your saliva duct is under your tongue, right behind your lower front teeth. Every four seconds, fresh saliva flows in the gully under your tongue. During an active kiss, your saliva flows more aggressively.

You need to pay attention to the amount of saliva that fills your mouth and swallow more frequently. Otherwise you soak your partner's mouth and yours too. This is NOT SEXY, nor is it appealing. A GREAT KISSER masters his/her kissing technique by remembering to monitor the flow of saliva. Even when babies drool, it is not thought of as "cute" by most people! It is definitely not cute for an adult to do so.

Exciting Pressure: You may like a firm, hard pressure against your mouth, but that does not mean you are with a partner that does. Or your partner might not like a feathery, light pressure either. One misinterpretation that more men have is the notion that women prefer very light kisses to firm, heavy pressured ones. It varies a great deal, and from all of the volunteers I worked with, we came away with the understanding that the choice did not follow any pattern. There were men that preferred a gentle kiss, as much as there were women that liked a rough embrace.

Our conclusion was that you CAN NOT generalize. You use the direct approach and simple ask: "Do you like a firm kiss more than a gentle, light kiss?" Be prepared for your partner to answer that question with "both" as their response. Most all of my volunteers liked both, depending on the situation that the kiss was occurring. However, three-quarters of them did have a preference to one over the other. For a passionate kiss, the firm kiss was more popular.

Ninety percent of my volunteers would prefer to have their partner try both styles with them, rather than asking the question, "what kind of kiss to you prefer?". It was their opinion that the kisses could be equally enjoyable depending on the techniques used to execute them. CONFIDENCE was the key factor to making them feel that the kiss was enjoyable. They felt that if they could sense that their partner knew what kind of kiss was being offered, it made them respond more favorably to it, regardless to the level of pressure being used.

Letting Up For Air: Everyone agrees that a kiss is not enjoyable if you find yourself struggling to breath! This may sound preposterous, but a lot of people close their partner's nostrils with their own anatomy (lips, cheeks, and nose). It may sound romantic to "take your partner's breath away", but if it happens for real, it is just uncomfortable.

Many people have no choice but to breathe out of their mouths. For these people, it is particularly important to let them "come up for air". Nothing can kill a romantic atmosphere, like an anxiety attack brought on by not getting enough air.

Unleashing The Fire In Your Partner's Body: There are very few people that do not enjoy a massage. Having one done with your tongue and lips is quite a sensual treat. The tongue is covered with sensory pads, and they are able to detect the tiniest nerve response. The intimacy of the contact heightens the reaction to the contact. Confidence becomes a problem for a lot of couples. Not a lack of confidence in the technique used, but in personal body image. The receiving partner may feel uncomfortable about their body. They may feel that their bodies are too lumpy, bumpy, or flabby. They might have scars or marks on their bodies that they are self-conscious about.

Here are some suggestions that will help: Soft lighting to be used for at least the first encounter. Candle lighting offers an additional aura for romantic responses. And use verbal affirmations to your partner that their body is attractive.

These are not the only elements to consider. Look them over, use them with your own partner, or perhaps they will open the dialogue for the two of you to make your own list. If I had the opportunity to have a list like this to work with my lover, perhaps it would have allowed our conversation to lead to a better conclusion.

Besides these ten, add creativity, flexibility and the desire to be in the company of your partner as important parts for a successful experience at becoming a "Great Kisser".

CHAPTER SIX

What a Great Kisser Does Next

As the title of this book indicates, great kissing leads to great sex. The problem that a lot of couples face is getting both people wanting to make love at the same time. The old phrases: "I have a headache", "Not now, I'm not in the mood", "Why don't you take a cold shower", and "Didn't we just have sex last week?" will forever go away, when you can get your partner's pheromones raging. Now you have the actual techniques down, you know what to do with your tongue, and lips. What's next?… there is so much more to becoming a great lover.

Communication is the key to any successful relationship and it certainly plays an integral part in kissing. You have to listen to your partner's verbal remarks, their non-verbal body language and know how to proceed. Ideally you want to match theirs with your own. Sometimes your interest will be put in front of your lovers and sometimes the reverse will happen. Part of communication is sharing. Both of you should feel comfortable to let the other one know where you want to go next. You might want to go from passionate kissing straight to making love. Your partner may or may not be ready to go to the full sexual act of intercourse. If you are truly a great lover, you will make certain that the pace towards intercourse is with a pace your partner is comfortable.

Letting your partner's needs exceed your own, is a sign of a great lover.

Performing the sensuous kiss that gets your partner in the mood to make love is what makes you a great lover. Our kissing method starts revving up your partner to want to make love just as much as you do!!! Using your lips to excite your partner's entire body is just the beginning…

Understanding Your Heart:

We all speak of "falling-in-love" as part of what our heart does for us. Being romantic is heart-felt. What you might not know is that the mechanical function of your heart truly does aide you in feeling sexy and making your lover feel sexy. Wherever your veins are close to the surface of your body, the nerve endings are particularly easy to entice. Here is the list of areas that are easy to reach and quick to arouse.

1. Temples
2. Ears
3. The carotid artery (on the sides of the neck)
4. Nipples (men and women)
5. Armpits
6. The inner side of the elbow bend
7. Wrists
8. Belly button (particularly an "innie")
9. Spine
10. The inner thigh
11. Behind the kneecaps
12. Fingertips and Toes

Some might find it fun to start at the top of your partner's head and work to their toes. Obviously the genitals are the one area that everyone knows are sensitive. But a truly great lover learns all the other parts of the body that can be turned on. Directing all your attention to your partner's crotch, keeps your love-making style predictable and sometimes boring.

Extending your tongue out of your mouth puts enough pressure on the muscle to make the tongue firm. This will allow you to put varying degrees of pressure on your partner's body. Using a "floppy" tongue will not offer much excitement. This is a story how one young man became a skillful lover with lessons about the body and massage.

Rondale was a twenty-six year old college graduate. He was raised in a small farm town in the Midwest. He had always wanted to get a professional massage. However in his small hometown, it was considered an open invitation to meet a prostitute. Clearly he grew up with limited understanding and appreciation for the tactile responses of his body. Then he went off to college in a fairly large city. During his senior year, the tension was so strong during mid-terms, that he sought out relief for his tired and knotted muscles. For a man that grew up as he had done, the decision to go to a massage salon was not an easy one to make. It would change his life in ways he could not have known ahead of his first appointment.

It was two o'clock on a Saturday afternoon, when Rondale hesitantly walked into the Stress Relief Center. The name of the salon should have made him more comfortable, but it did not effect him at all. The moment he walked inside, he heard new-wave music softly playing and the air had a smell of sweet jasmine. Rondale was not at all sure that this was a good idea. But he was too timid to cancel the appointment. And it turned out to be a great decision to stay where he was, waiting for his first massage. Then Miraeh greeted him with a gorgeous smile and firm double handed handshake. She guided him into the cubicle where his massage would take place.

The room was small but absolutely spotlessly clean. The room looked more like an examination room than a massage salon. This made Rondale much more at ease. Then Miraeh instructed him to remove all of his clothes and lay on the massage table, face up and he can lay the small towel over his genitals. She promptly left the room and dimmed the lights as she exited. Rondale was left to undress with great feelings of apprehension. But he did as he was instructed. Then Miraeh knocked softly on the door, and waited for Rondale to agree to let her enter. Not knowing what he should do or what he was going to experience, he laid there very nervously. Miraeh did not speak, she just went to work mixing some solutions from a series of clear containers. The smells that permeated the air told Rondale that she was making a concoction was very light but not too flowery. He couldn't identify the fragrance, but it reminded him of a musk like scent. As Miraeh touched his face, her fingers told him that she knew what she was going. He didn't spend any time thinking about her or whether or not if she was capable to do this massage. Now he couldn't help but bring all of his attention to what she was doing to his body. It was as if his body had taken over his brain, the sensations were so strong. Nerve endings he never knew he had became alive. His entire body tingled and goose-flesh developed where ever Miraeh's fingers moved.

The massage lasted an hour, but for Rondale it could not be long enough. Rondale became Miraeh's most regular client. For the rest of his senior year he never missed an appointment.

Nothing got in the way of his massage. Rotten weather, or the need to study for an exam did NOT force him to cancel a single session.

What developed between Miraeh and Rondale was also unexpected by both of them. They fell in love. The massage session then became very personal, and done in their own apartment. If Rondale thought he knew what his body could feel like during a massage, Miraeh was soon to teach him more about his body than he ever thought possible. After six months, Rondale learned about the intense response his body gave him as Miraeh moved over his skin. But now that she was responding to Rondale as a lover, she did not approach his body as a clinical masseuse. She used her lips to entice his body. Miraeh explained in detail how to manipulate the surface of the skin to obtain the intense sensations. Within a few lessons, Rondale was then able to perform similar massage movements on Miraeh. From that moment on, Rondale became a very skilled lover.

Ironically, Rondale had previously thought of himself as a very talented lover. He had not heard any of his previous lovers complain about his techniques, so he was not looking to change his approach. Miraeh had changed all that. If he could, he would have retraced his path with past lovers to show them what he now knew how to do to excite and give sexual pleasure. That was not very likely to happen, but his future lovers would certainly get first hand experience in his "full-body lip/mouth" massages....

CHAPTER SEVEN

When to Reach for a Mint(Halitosis)

The actual condition is more than having bad breath. Although bad breath is a clear definitive sign of the problem. It is created due to several factors. The level of bacteria in the mouth is too high. The bacteria causes certain gasses to form in the saliva, and the soft tissue inside of the mouth and gums. These gasses give off an offensive smell.

Behind your lower two front teeth lies one of the major saliva ducts of your mouth. From this duct, fresh saliva is secreted into your mouth, every four seconds. Your saliva is clear, it has a high acid pH to attack the food you eat, and has little taste or smell. It is the first part of the digestion system. The enzymatic breakdown of your food starts in your mouth with the use of the saliva. At least that is the basic characteristics for healthy saliva. When you swallow, the mouth is rinsed with fresh saliva.

The bacteria clings to the tongue, the soft tissue of the mouth, and gums. It mixes in with the saliva, and effects it's ability to breakdown food particles. The bacteria gasses and saliva mixture creates the foul smell, the condition called halitosis. The saliva is always renewing itself, but the bacteria grows just as quickly. The stomach acids breed the bacteria gasses that travel into the mouth.

A person would have to brush their teeth and tongue every twenty to thirty minutes to keep a handle on the level of bacteria that clings to their teeth, tongue and gums. Flossing around the gum line of the teeth would have to be done after each meal, rather than at the end of each day. But all of that will not kill the bacteria that is produced in the stomach. The condition needs medical attention. The patient will have to work closely with their dentist and nutritionist to gain total control of the condition. The doctor will often times prescribe drugs to kill the bacteria. While the nutritionist will work with the patient teaching them how to prepare their diet. The nutritionist will offer suggestions in what food groups are needed, as well as other ways to prepare the food that will reduce the bacteria count. A lot of the times, patients with chronic halitosis are put on restricted amounts of dairy foods. All dairy foods induce phlegm and mucus to develop in the mouth and stomach. Both contribute to the gasses and the smell of halitosis.

Popping in breath mints, like "Certs" is NOT a solution to the problem of halitosis, it simply helps to mask the odor of the condition. There are other products on the market that have been designed to aide in the reduction of halitosis, but are only mildly effective.

Having halitosis is problem that is far more intense than disrupting a great kiss. It does need constant work and care to get it under control. However during the interim, a person can take the following precautionary measures to reduce the negative feedback that is sure to come up during a long and romantic kiss.

1. Plan carefully the foods you are going to eat the day that you plan on having a romantic interlude. Make sure they are not going to contribute to the smells in your mouth. The following

is just a small list of foods that are known to increase the smells caught in your mouth:

Garlic, Onions, Raw sprouts, Deep Fried Foods, Yogurt, Soft-served frozen yogurt, Chili, Raw Broccoli or Cauliflower, Brussels sprouts, and Cabbage.

2. Always carry toothpaste, mouthwash and a toothbrush with you everywhere you go.

3. Remember to floss after every meal. This includes the meal you will be sharing with your partner. At the end of dinner, get to a bathroom and quickly floss then brush, and rinse with mouthwash. Your partner will be impressed with your commitment to good oral hygiene.

4. Carry small breath mints with you at all times.

** Beware that keeping candy style breath fresheners can have a direct effect on the enamel of your teeth. Sugar-based candy can cause the a breakdown of the teeth. Check with your dentist for suggestions in handling your desire for fresh breath while keeping your teeth free from attack.

5. During the time you are actually kissing, make sure that you swallow frequently. Pay attention to how much saliva builds in your mouth during the kiss and try to not pass it on to your partner.

Whether you have a problem with halitosis or any mild bad breath problem, you should pay attention to the amount of saliva that builds inside of your mouth during kissing. It is not inviting to have your partner get a mouth full of your saliva!!!

CHAPTER EIGHT

You Are No Longer a Baby— So Why Are You Still Drooling?

When you were teething it was expected that you would be always drooling all over yourself and anyone else too. As an adult it is not cool to drool. In men, the triggering of pheromones is directly effecting their saliva releases. As part of nature, it has been said that the male calls out to it's mate. Perhaps the increase in saliva is to allow the male to get their throats ready for the "mating call". Regardless as to the reasons why men get a mouth full of saliva when they get aroused, they must be more careful to SWALLOW BEFORE they approach their partner's mouth! When pheromones are released into the body they have a different reaction on males than on females. From my group of women, we all agreed that our mouths were drier then the men we kissed.

Nothing is more annoying than having a mouthful of saliva dumped into the other's mouth during a kiss. You have to be aware to make sure yours or your partner's saliva DOES NOT pour into the other's mouth. Besides being very uncomfortable, it also is the fastest way to get sick. All saliva has bacteria in it and when another person's saliva mixes with your own it changes your body's balance of bacteria. It is the fastest way to develop a cold, a sore throat or both. It also GREATLY REDUCES the chances that the kiss will feel sensual, and make you feel romantic.

In extolling all the sensual virtues of Sensual Kissing, certain health risks were not mentioned. But they do exist, you have to be careful of mouth ulcers. Although a mouth ulcer is part of the herpes virus family, it is not an STD. It is never-the-less, contagious. If either partner has a mouth ulcer in the soft tissue of their gums, the viral spores will be passed to the other partner through Sensual Kissing. It is usually difficult to directly ask your partner before you kiss, "Do you have any mouth ulcers?" Learning about your partner's health is still important.

What makes it even more difficult, is the increase in herpes simplex II in the mouth due to an increase in oral sex. Both of these herpes look exactly the same. Both have the concave indents, with white pus filled in the hole. Both will be painful at first, and then as they begin to heal they are significantly less painful. Some will not hurt at all. As tough as it is, you still you have to ask the difficult questions. Without taking the time to ask, you are placing yourself in great risk from exposing your mouth to an STD (sexually transmitted disease). If there are any signs of an ulcer or herpes outbreak on the edges of the lips, it is important to keep your distance. If either partner has any active breakouts in their mouth and then they perform oral sex on the other, the transfer of the virus to the genitals is highly possible.

I realize that this issue is difficult to bring up, particularly in casual dating. Even the most casual meeting can turn into a passionate embrace sometime during the evening. Under these circumstances, it is not very likely that medical information will be exchanged. Ideally it would advisable to keep Sensual Kissing to relationships that have more concrete substance to them. Ironically, once you master Sensual Kissing, the typical closed mouth kiss will seem uninteresting. You are left feeling like you have been placed between a "rock and a hard place".

Upon careful consideration of this issue, the participants were asked to offer some suggestions as to how to deal with a passionate embrace with a very new-acquaintance, and the risk of herpes or a mouth ulcer. Here are their replies:

1. Try to look over the partner's mouth, lips, teeth and gums while they talk. Without looking like you are searching for anything specific, try to pay attention to the conditions around their mouth.

2. IF it can be worked into the conversation, bring up your dentist, a commercial for some special toothpaste or dental product. Get them to reveal as much about dental care as possible.

3. Should the first encounter include a meal, make sure you make a point to brush your teeth afterwards. Add into your conversation the interest you have for good oral hygiene. Watch their reaction to your comments.

4. Whenever possible keep the kissing to a less intense level until you know more about your partner's health situation.

Everyone agreed it would terrific if they could just come out and say "In these challenging times, it's important to know about herpes and other STD's, have you had any experiences I should know about?". Although everyone thought it was important, we all agreed it is VERY DIFFI-CULT to execute such a line of conversation when all you are doing is casual kissing. The entire group agreed that if any sexual contact is to take place, these questions MUST be clarified. Embarrassing or not, your life is just to precious to be put at such a high risk. AIDS has changed the way we relate to casual sex forever.

CHAPTER NINE

Braces and Romance

We can all remember the trials and tribulations of being a pre-teen with a full set of braces on our teeth. Many nights we would lay in our beds worrying what our friends would say to the metal "railroad tracks"

> "Would we ever be invited to the boy-girl parties while the braces were on our teeth?"
>
> "Could we expect a goodnight kiss at the end of the school dance?"
>
> "If two kids with braces kissed, would the braces get caught and tangled together?"

As the baby-boomer generation grew up and created a new power-driven professional working style, their appearances became important enough to re-evaluate the need for perfect teeth.

Adding to their decision was the improved technologies in orthodontics, which put the "railroad track" phenomenon to rest. The newer versions have created a trend in orthodontics, that has allowed anyone to obtain braces. The technology has progressed so far that the largest group having braces on their teeth are 35-45 year olds.

With adults getting full-set braces for business reasons, they still have to deal with the personal and social ramifications of their decision. The braces are better looking, smaller in size, and a lot less imposing on the teeth. However, they are still NOT considered "sexy". As adults, the baby-boomers are interacting with adults in a more sexual fashion than the pre-teens ever would. (I must regrettably admit that sexual exploration is getting to be a way of life in pre-teen ages too.) The person wearing the braces will have to adjust their kissing style to accommodate the braces.

Of those interviewed, about 25% had personal experiences with braces. Less than ten percent (9.1%) actually wore braces as an adult. The level of interest in sensual kissing and braces was directly influenced on who was actually wearing the braces.

With the question: Would you hesitate to offer a sensual kiss to some-one wearing braces? Here are their answers. The 9.1% did not have any hesitation. They just felt that they would cover their teeth with their lips. The others felt that sensual kissing did not hold a high level of interest. Several men showed hesitation to kiss at all if their partners wore braces. The women stated that the men showing hesitation, were concerned that the braces would cut the soft tissue of their bottom lip. The women also stated that new relationships were more bothered by the braces than long-term ones.

Not only are braces part of our Baby Boomer Generation, the Internet and e-mail has created new ways to complicate the dating scene. Here's just one woman's experience:

> Marlene had met Neal through a chat room on AOL. She had begun to use the Internet for a research project at work. Then she got hooked on the freedom that the chat rooms provided and found herself logging 20 hours a week on her computer's AOL line. Marlene had not found going to bars or other hang-out clubs very enjoyable. All the things that made her nervous

and anxious in public were not an issue in the privacy of her home. Being over forty and wearing a full mouth of braces was just one of many reasons she felt self-conscious. Although the braces were necessary to correct her jaw-line as well as her teeth, she still hated how they made her look. Through long nights at each other's terminals, Neal and Marlene typed out details about their lives. After three months of this nightly ritual, they agreed to meet.

Since Neal did not ask Marlene to describe what she looked like, nor did they exchange photographs during their intense cybernetic courtship, Marlene never brought up the fact that she was wearing full railroad tracks. Even though there were much newer style braces, her condition required the old-fashion metal fittings over all of her teeth. The night finally came when they would meet face-to-face. They decided to meet at a local bar. Marlene thought the crowds and dim lighting would work to her advantage. Neal had his own self-doubts going through his head. What he had not conveyed to her through the lengthy written dialogues was that he was only five feet two.

Marlene recalls sitting at a corner table with butterflies in her stomach and sweaty palms. Neal was fighting his own case of the jitters. But the minute their eyes locked, they knew that their fears were all for naught. Her braces were not a problem, nor was the fact that Marlene was seven inches taller than Neal when he was wearing his platform shoes. The chemistry was there, even more than when they would log on their computers, and be able to finish each other's sentences.

Previously I described playful ways to tug on your partner's lips and gums to entice and sexual turn them on. When wearing braces, it is not easily performed. Perhaps not able to be done at all. Of the group wearing braces, most said that at first they refrained from even trying to do much kissing. They mentioned that their teeth and gums were very tender and sore. This pain and discomfort reduced their interest in kissing for several weeks, some even months.

> Neal had commented that he was the aggressor when it came to kissing. Although Marlene seemed to enjoy him kissing her, she didn't initiate any of the kissing. For a while it did not bother him. As their relationship grew over time, it did make him wonder. Marlene, on the other hand, still felt uneasy about what she could or couldn't do with all the metal in her mouth. She didn't think she could ask her orthodontist about it, and she didn't have any other friends that were going through it themselves.

> Finally Neal just came out and asked her why she didn't just come out and plant a big fat kiss on him? Sheepishly she tried to explain her hesitation about her braces. Neal was very good about it and just said it didn't make him feel less interested in kissing her. After that conversation, Marlene couldn't wait to greet him every day with a long passionate kiss…

Many people notice an increase in breath odor. This could be contributed to the new way they have to brush their teeth. Regardless, their breath was not as fresh as before the braces. This also added to their hesitation with passionate kissing. (Certainly wasn't Marlene's experience.)

Other forms of sex were definitely effected. The scope of these book will not get into these areas.

CHAPTER TEN

Cuddling and Cooing

If you have ever been put into the awkward situation like these women you can understand the value of knowing the secrets of the sensuous kiss.

While most people can not wait for Friday to be over, in anticipation of Saturday morning, Annette dreaded it. She awoke to every Saturday morning with her 264 pound husband mounting her for a "quickie". In less than ten minutes, he gave her a peck on the cheek, a "you are the greatest" and rolled over happy and content while she rushed to the bathroom to hide her tears with the sound of the water running in the sink.

She began to dread her Saturday mornings so much she actually tried to get out of bed before her husband woke up just so as to avoid the "Saturday Special". That's what he called it, although her view of it was anything but special. Annette longed for the days and nights when they first started to date. They would kiss for hours and hours. She remembered coming in from their dates with her lips "on fire" and the rest

of her body tingling and excited. Oh how she would love to go back into time…

When I met Annette and she shared with me this situation, I suggested that the moment that she awakened by the weight of her husband on top of her, that she initiates a sensual kiss. Give her husband something to jar his memory of their necking sessions. With a great deal of intrepidation, she agreed to try it.

I saw Annette seven weeks later, and asked her "How were things going?" Her smile told me the answer as she said: "Saturday Specials" have turned into "Friday nights and Saturday mornings". She said her husband was so surprised at first, which he had no idea that she was so unhappy about the way the weekends started. He did not want them to be like so many other couples he had heard about that stopped reaching out for the other, after so many years of marriage. He was under the impression that he was pleasing her and himself with the way he would awaken her each Saturday. With the proper communication, and the help of sensual kissing, they are keeping the magic in their relationship.

Deanna had a different kind of challenge that she shared with me. Her boyfriend loved to set the alarm a half an hour early just so they had a full thirty minutes to cuddle before they started their day. She was uncomfortable with "morning mouth" and passionate kissing. Deanna just could not get comfortable with it. Popping out of bed to brush her teeth and then trying to "recapture" the spontaneity was not working either. She shared her frustration with me and I suggested the following two ideas. One worked better than the other. Here are what my ideas were:

> I suggested to keep some thin mints in the night stand next to her side of the bed. Then she could reach for one and instead of just popping it into her mouth and rolling it around to get rid of her "morning mouth", she could place it between her

front teeth and offer to share half of it with her boyfriend. By the method of sharing of the mint between the two of them, Deanna would keep the spontaneity of the morning going and still feel more comfortable with her breath.

Another method of ridding yourself of morning breath is to have a breath spray in easy reach. Deanna could take a second and spray before she turned to face her partner. She tried this idea first, but the sound of the spray broke the magic of the moment for her boyfriend. He liked the idea of them coming together for the first kiss, and the having the tiny mint to play with between the two of them. They made it a game. Whenever either of them found unique flavors of small mints or candies they could not wait to surprise the other with the new taste the next morning.

For a lot of people cuddling is a message that everything is all right between them. Non-verbal messages seem to be less demanding,and usually far less confrontational. Using cuddling as a way to keep the connection between you strong and loving can always be aided by wonderful sensual kissing. Remember that sex does not always have to be part of sensual kissing. Just enjoying the closeness and the touching of the two of you, can be the sole purpose of the experience. No matter what the reasons, do not let another day or night go by without at least one sensual kiss. Now you have the knowledge and confidence of "**Pucker Power**". You are now a master of the perfect sensuous kiss!

A few words about Part One… From The Author:

I have written Part One of "Pucker Power" for your enjoyment. It was never my intent to present this information as the only way to perform sensual kissing. We will all have our own special methods and ideas, as we should. However, I spent more than ten years exploring this topic with many, many friends and associates. Together we decided that there really needed to be some clear definite techniques put to paper. And so with that in mind, Pucker Power was created. I sincerely hope that you will play with the ideas presented. Take from them what you like and find yourself in endless hours of exploration and enjoyment. Whether you are married to the love of your life, or still seeking to find the right partner to spend your days with, may Pucker Power be part of your happy, sensual experiences.

With Love,

Shelley

PART TWO

A woman's journey into dating and Pucker Power is put to the test......

A few comments FROM THE AUTHOR:

I wrote this section of the book for the sheer enjoyment of being able to share the stories with you. I was blessed with the opportunity to share all the situations with my friends, family and my special clients. After each experience was completed, they said I should have written it down. It was my desire to offer humor to the reader through my experiences.

For legal protection, I have changed the names of everyone. Besides, I did not want to get anyone upset at my disclosure of private moments. As you would soon read, many were far from private…

But they were funny. Many people would be able to relate to the events that happened to me while dating. When going through it, the situation sometimes lacked humor, then later it made me laugh.

CHAPTER ELEVEN

First Dates

Story One: First Dates and Movies

I was always surprised how many times "going to a movie" was suggested as the first date. If you were set up on a blind date, the protection of the dark theater could have provided solace if your date turned out to be more *nerdy* than *hunky*. What was the attraction of being silent with each other for two hours while the action on the silver screen was all that kept you together?

When you first met, finding something to talk about should not have been a problem. Better yet, if it was a problem you should know early on, so that both could have moved on and not struggled with the awkwardness. The media had convinced me that good communication was essential for a successful relationship. Therefore, if no communication existed, I would not have wanted to drag out the inevitable....which was the break up.

With that said, I have had many movie dates. While we watched some romantic movie, I often wondered if my date was having any ideas to

repeat some sexual scene that was being acted out. Of course the participants could have been two great looking actors, like Mel Gibson and
Michelle Pfiefer Then I began to think of all the ways I was never going
to look like Michelle. Somehow the fact that my date was never going to
look like Mel didn't seem as important. (If you ask one hundred women
if they are pretty, 81% of them will mention about some feature or flaw
in their appearance. * Ask one hundred men if they are handsome and
98% will answer Yes. Why, because the alternative is not even a consideration for them. *Ladies*, we need to take lessons from them on this one
issue. *(Taken from a poll in ***Cosmopolitan Magazine***.)

Often when I would walk into a dark movie theater, I would remember
a memory of my dating in high school. I grew up in Baltimore. The
movie theaters had balconies then. And the back rows were the prime
location where all the *hot lovers* sat. Back then, when a first date went for
those seats, I knew I was in for the "octopus-tango". I also knew that the
date would be a short one…

Now as an adult in Southern California, I have found that some things
have changed while others have stayed the same. This brought to mind
my first date with Mo. I met him while at my bank, during a break in my
appointments at the salon. Like many small business operators, I
banked at the branch in the shopping center where my salon was
located. I was wearing my traditional lab coat over my normal clothes.
On that afternoon, I was deep in thought while waiting in line and did
not notice anyone else in line. It was probably just as well, because if I
had noticed Mo checking me out, I probably would have felt self-conscious. Since I was wearing my name tag on my lab coat, it was easier for
Mo as he started up a conversation with me. He seemed nice enough. IF
first impressions were any indicator, he appeared to be a blue collar
worker. He wore blue jeans and a white shirt, opened at the collar and
no tie. His sleeves were rolled up, and his biceps were well defined. His
skin was weather-beaten and his eyes crinkled at the ends when he

smiled. I definitely liked his smile: it was broad and warm. His blond hair had had way too much sun exposure, and his eyes were crystal blue. I guessed his age to be about 38. Being in the skin care business, my guesses were often close to bulls-eye. In less than ten minutes, he had asked me out and I decided to say yes. I was going to have a long night with clients but the following evening I was available. And so we did. Unfortunately, he immediately suggested a *movie*. I was very disappointed at his lack of creativity. But said nothing other than OK. And so our first date was to go see the movie "**An Officer and a Gentlemen**". I offered to meet him at the theater. He insisted that he pick me up at my home. I took that as a sign of a well mannered man. We set the time for seven pm. and to my surprise he was just a few minutes early. I decided to stay in the dress I was wearing during the day. Since I had my lab coat on all day, it wasn't dirty. To appear more casual, I removed my jewelry and brushed my hair down my back. For work, I kept it in a chignon. That style was not very sexy, but practical that kept my hair from falling into my clients' faces. Wearing it down seemed to be more appealing to men. I must have made the right decision, because Mo commented on how long my hair was. In the bank he had thought I had short hair, but said he preferred women with long hair. I thought that was supposed to be compliment. And took it as such.

The movie theater was all of ten minutes away, but Mo drove like a bat-out-of-hell. I was grateful that I had followed the law and had buckled my seatbelt. I was sure that I would fall to the floor if I hadn't. We drove on side streets and yet his speedometer still read over 50 mph. There wasn't a line for tickets so we had over half an hour to wait for the movie to start. I suggested that we go to a near by coffee shop. Mo rejected my idea and wanted to stand outside of the theater till the show started. It was an incredibly long thirty minutes. Conversation was usually one of my strong points. Our problem came from not having any common interests. Lucky for me, Mo was the kind of guy that loved to talk about himself without asking any questions about anyone else. He grew up on a farm in Idaho and had six brothers and one sister. He was one of the middle children, but was not clear on exactly where in line he fell. No one in his family went to college and he wouldn't have finished high school, except for a GED he received in the army. When he got out, he used the GI bill and got his license in electrician school. Someday he planned to have his own electrician shop. I had been right about his age, he was 38. Born a Gemini, although I never knew what that really was supposed to have told me. Those astrology charts were difficult to follow. Anyway, it was clear that we came from totally different backgrounds. And our opinions about education couldn't have been more opposite.

Finally the time was up and the movie was ready to start. He wanted to sit in the very last rows. At first I was going to agree and then I decided that a few seats away from the last row was probably safer....Reluctantly, Mo agreed that two seats in the middle of the third row from the last would be acceptable. Mo sat there with one arm pinning my shoulders to the back of the chair, while he clasped my right hand into his sweaty palm. Too bad our hands were not preoccupied with any concession snacks. I could have had a reason to get my hand back without hurting his feelings. He hadn't asked if I wanted any refreshments. Initially I thought it might have been for financial reasons. And being a woman affected by the 90's concept of dating, I offered to buy some popcorn and sodas too. He immediately responded with how he hated the sounds of crunching and slurping during the movie. That resolved my money theory. With a stiff neck and squirmish palm, I tried to enjoy a well acted, and dramatic story line. As Deborah Winger was being carried through the factory at the end of the movie, Mo leaned over and said in a voice that seemed like it was coming through a microphone "Shel baby, wouldn't you like me to pick you up and carry you to bed tonight?" I wanted the floor to open up and bury me on the spot!!! This was our first date, and if there had been even a tiny chance for a second, that comment ended it. It's hard to put me at a loss of words....the only ones that came to mind at that moment were not very lady-like and so I sat dumb-founded. I prayed that the whole theater had not heard him. I was certain that the people on either side, back, and front of me, probably had. If looks could have killed, mine would have at least caused him some major distress!

I could not wait to get back to the car. There I could have at least said something without adding to my embarrassment. But alas, Mo had to continue his tirade while we walked out of the movie. "Hon, that was great": he said. That movie had put him in the mood for sex. He wanted to go to his place, it was closer to the theater.

I had had enough; I could not have gone on another moment. By all means I thought he should have gone home immediately. I would have been happy to call it a night and called a cab to get home. Mo didn't believe I hadn't eagerly accepted and jumped into his bed.... He stood there a moment and then his final statement put final closure to the real-time nightmare. "You ungrateful bitch!" he yelled. Since he had sprung for the movie and had considered taking me for coffee and pie afterwards, I was supposed to be compliant to his demands.

I walked to the box office and called for a cab.

Many months later I happened to run into Mo and his date at another movie. I suddenly wondered what her opinion of him might have been. I was to get my answer sooner than expected. While I was in the ladies room, she walked in and ran to the sink to wash her hands. She looked so upset, I felt sorry for her. I went up to her and said "Excuse me, I couldn't have helped noticing you came in with Mo". She had a shocked look on her face, as she replied "Oh my G-d, you know him?" Sadly I said: "One and only one date with him several months ago. We had gone to see "**An Officer and A Gentlemen**" and I ended up taking a cab home." She said that if she had enough money for the fare, she would have gotten one just then. I felt so bad for her, I offered to give her a lift home if she really needed one. She said she did.

One good thing Mo did for us, he created two good friends. Years later, if I saw "**An Officer and A Gentlemen**", I would break up laughing.

Story Two: Match-Making at 35,000 Feet

There are two opposing clichés that I have had difficulty deciding how to work into my life. The first one states: "You must look for love", and the other one states: " Love comes when you least expect it. Finally I decided to combine these two concepts. I would not have actively tried to find a man, but would not have turned down any opportunity to meet someone either.

I tried to make sure that my makeup, hair, nails and clothes were always presentable no matter where or when I went out. This included grocery shopping, car washes, or gas stations. So it was no surprise that I tried to "Put On My Best Face" when I traveled to Atlanta to lecture. (I wrote the Internationally successful makeup series *"PUTTING YOUR BEST FACE FORWARD*™"

I never knew who would be seated next to me on the plane. I would be so excited if any airline included the opportunity to select the type of passenger you would be seated next to. I could imagine how that process would have increased the public's interest in flying if the ticket reservationist would ask: "Did you want an isle or window seat next to a woman, or man? or "Would you like a married or single person seated next to you?" Mothers with small children could all be seated together, the married wives could have had someone to relate too, and the single passengers could have traveled with someone that they could have flirted with or at least shared similar experiences.

On this flight to Atlanta, I was seated next to a very chatty woman who could not get over the size of my makeup case. As a holistic skin care and makeup artist, I needed to make certain that my cosmetics arrived with me on any flight. Therefore, I wouldn't have checked this case with the baggage handlers. She spent the full five hours picking my brain about skin care and makeup tips. Too bad I could not have charged her a consultation fee...we parted in friendly fashion. Just in case she ever needed the services of a facialist while in Orange County, CA., I gave her my business card.

A week after my return, I got a phone call from a man named Joe. He had gotten my number from this woman. Based on whatever this woman had told him, Joe was under the impression that we should have gone out on a date. Although I was initially taken by complete surprise, I thought what would I really have to lose?... (Remember I attempted to keep the clichés in mind.) I continued to speak to him for forty minutes. It was crystal clear that we had absolutely **nothing** in common. I didn't understand how this woman thought we were such a good match. By the end of the conversation, it was apparent to me that the **only common ground** we had was ....**we were both single**. Perhaps to some people, that was all it took. Here's how I interpreted our differences:

Joe	Shelley
Married 20 yrs. w/4 kids	Never married but was in a 12 yr. relationship
Blamed his ex for everything	Still was friendly with my ex
Salesman for a company	Business owner for 12 yrs.
HS graduate—hated school and reading	2 masters degrees, author of 8 books

Loved camping, hiking and sports	Loved reading, theater, and music
Traveled very little	Traveled on a National lecture tour

We got off the phone with the possibility of connecting after my return from my second speaking engagement in Washington DC. I really thought that I would not hear from him again. It was obvious that we hadn't made much of a connection on the first phone call.

Then two months later on a Friday night, I picked up the phone to hear Joe's voice. He knew he had said he would call when I returned from DC. He said that based on the new book "**The Rules**" a woman was not supposed to accept a last minute invitation. However, he had just been given two tickets to see Barbara Mandrell, the next night. He remembered that I liked country western music and asked if I would like to go?.

Truthfully I was impressed that he read the book, although I hated it. He even remembered what music I liked. I gladly accepted the date. (it turns out he heard about the book on some talk show and had not personally read it.)

He told me that the concert was somewhere in Orange County. Since he lived in LA, I offered to meet him, and he said he would prefer to pick me up if I felt safe enough to give him my address. Again I was impressed with his thoughtfulness, and gave him directions. Joe said it started at 8:00 p.m. and would pick me up at 7:15 p.m. I decided that this meant that going out to dinner was not to be part of the date. That was OK with me, I would have preferred to eat at home. I got off of the phone before I realized that I had not asked exactly where the concert was to be held.

I called Ticket masters and they said that Ms Mandrell would be at the Performing Arts Center along with the Pacific Symphony Orchestra. So much for real down home country music. I happened to love classical music just as much. I knew that the Performing Arts Center was very classy, and that people dressed up to go there, particularly on a Saturday night. I got dressed that evening in a black, short, velvet cocktail dress and diamond accessories. Then Joe called at 6:45 p.m. saying that he just got home from a game and would shower and be right over....From LA??? He mentioned that I had never said what I looked like. I just figured that the woman from the plane had filled him in on those details. I had not asked him what he looked like either. As much as my presentation meant a lot to me, I did not care that much what he looked like. I decided to describe what I would be wearing and an overview of my general appearance. I considered myself *"Very cosmetically prepared, 5'2", but not petite*—another way of saying I am NOT thin, *long wavy auburn hair and large expressive eyes with a warm smile."* Then I told him what I would be wearing. Joe immediately offered his opinion of the concert. He said it would be very casual and that he would wear jeans, a shirt and cowboy boots". He said he liked very short skirts and asked if I owned any? I then rushed to change into a country style short skirt, jacket, boots and matching cowgirl hat. Of course, off went the diamonds. He was glad that I was short, since he was 5'7" and didn't like women taller than him.

He arrived at 7:20 p.m.. After I described myself to him, he flew down to see me. He said: "You did not do yourself justice." According to Joe, this woman had not said anything about what I looked like when she first suggested that he call. Joe was 5'7" if he were wearing lifts in his boots, he had a pounchy face with a bulbous nose. He wore faded blue jeans that had one tiny hole on the left knee, a blue and red checker shirt, and brown cowboy boots. His stomach hung so much over his black belt, with a huge bulls head buckle that he could have been carrying a baby inside of his denim shirt. I was not excited by his appearance but I was not unhappy either.

We arrived at the concert minutes before it started, but many people were still lingering in the lobby with drinks and hors d'ouvres. I noticed all eyes were on us. NOT because we were late, but because they were all in sequins dresses, evening gowns, tuxedoes and suits. Joe and I looked like hay-seeds and I wished the ground had gobbled us both up. Joe seemed not to notice. Wish I could have said the same, maybe it's a woman's thing. I said nothing, as he walked up to the bar and ordered a beer. "Did you want one?" he called over to me. I said I would take a soda. The bartender started to pour the beer in a glass, when Joe tried to stop him. He preferred to drink it from the bottle. The bartender attempted to explain that all drinks had to be poured. When Joe insisted, the bartender poured my drink and asked for $6.00. Joe gave him exact change. I thought about slipping a dollar into the tip jar. It stood right in front of us, but I decided it was better manners to leave well enough alone. We proceed to our seats with our drinks. I considered mentioning that we would probably not be allowed in with the drinks. Just then a security person stopped us and said that we would have to return to the lobby with our drinks. So much for my attempt at being subtle, we were really getting noticed now. The stares were getting stronger. Joe chug-a-lugged his beer, and I just tossed my soda. I could not wait to get to our seats where it would be somewhat dark and I could enjoy the entertainment. Joe took my hat and placed it on the seat next to him. I thought it was a kind gesture.

Then he proceeded to speak into my ear and twirled my hair. His voice was not soft, his breath reeked, and my hair felt like it was being twisted into a mesh of knots. Someone behind us asked him to be quiet, and I was *grateful*. Then came the pinning of my shoulders and neck with his arm and as he grabbed my hand with his sweaty palm. How was it I seemed to be so lucky to find these men??? **Maybe women just have dry palms and men are supposed to have sweaty ones......**

The concert was fantastic. The Pacific Symphony Orchestra was the opening act and played a medley of Gershwin and Berlin tunes. I really enjoyed the blend of orchestra and Barbara Mandrell's performance. Ms. Mandrell had sung, danced, and played five instruments. She never left the stage, not even to make three costume changes. Her energy level would have gone off of the charts if we could have gauged it. After a fabulous show like that one, I was so energized and excited. I only wished I was born with some kind of musical talent…

Joe was greatly disappointed. He had not liked the PSO at all. And he thought Barbara's choices of songs were not "country enough". He thought she had crossed over to "pop music". Quite frankly, I hadn't noticed. As we walked back to the car, I wondered if he would suggest going for coffee. I decided where we might go to continue the date. He had made it clear he was totally unfamiliar with the area. He seemed deep in thought. I was mildly curious as to what might be preoccupying his mind. I soon found out…

He did not remember where he had parked the car. Joe became irate and thought I should have remembered. I usually did not pay any attention unless I was driving. After twenty minutes we finally found the car. Joe was still mad and said that we should go back to my place to chat and *get to know one another better*. My internal alarm began to flash, "what exactly was on his mind?" I kept the conversation light, as we approached my street.

Inside my apartment, he asked if I had anything to drink. Luckily, I had a chilled bottle of white wine. Although I never drank, I tried to keep a bottle of wine in the refrigerator for moments just like that one. I gave him the cork screw and poured some soda, for myself. He was unable to use the cork screw and said that his bottles came without a cork. I managed to get the bottle open and we sat on the couch. We both kicked off our shoes. The conversation went smoothly. However, it became even clearer that we had no common reference points at all!! It was now almost 2 am., Joe had managed to polish off ¾'s of the bottle, he was obviously intoxicated and I suggested that I call him a cab. He responded: "Hell no, I've driven more smashed than this." IF this was supposed to relieve my mind, it did not. I tried to persuade him to let me call someone. He refused. As I walked him to the door, he reached out and gave me a big hug. In seconds, it was obvious that he was fully erect, and he said: "Well you've given me a woody, wanna fool around?" I broke away and gently pushed him out of the door. I did not know whether I prayed to fall asleep to try to forget that evening or feared that it would be relived all night, in a nightmare....

Story Three: Cat and Mouse

Although I would have been the first to admit that some games adults play were not very wise, this was one that really could have saved my life. Ever since I was an infant, I had a strange, overwhelming reaction to moving vehicles. Train, plane, boat, bus, or car it did not matter, if it had a vibration to it, I would have fallen asleep in it. Once I turned sixteen and a licensed driver, I had to find a way to break the reaction. The cat and mouse game solved my initial problem. The game was simple. Two drivers in two separate cars would pattern their driving in a tag-like style. One drove a bit ahead of the other and then the rear driver came along side of the front car and "tagged" the driver with a nod of their head. The second driver then attempted to take the lead. This forced the other driver to chase and catch up and "tag" again.

On my way home from work on September 12, 1983 I was in a particularly good mood. I had had a great day in the salon. I had my hair done during the day, and was planning to meet my best friend for Happy Hour at our favorite restaurant. It was to be a long night. After the socializing was over, I was going home to cook my special chicken dish for the entire staff for lunch the next day. Therefore, I decided to keep awake on the long ride home by playing the game with someone on the freeway. Soon after getting on the 55 freeway, I spotted a charming-looking man in a small sports car. I finally matched his stride and motioned as I began the game. The man in a black Austin Martin seemed agreeable.

We had been going for several miles on the 55 freeway, and I was the lead car. All of the sudden I sensed he was coming up onto my passenger side of my silver Mazda GLC. He was very cute and so I decided to flash him a flirtatious smile. Much to my surprise it was a *different* man altogether!! Boy was I embarrassed. That man was driving a black Porsche. He appeared to be thin, had short, brown hair and was wearing a blue, long sleeved shirt and red tie. The smile and suggestive wink I had just sent over to him, left little to the imagination. Now what was I going to do?? The man in the Austin Martin was nowhere to be seen. Perhaps he saw what had happened and decided to cut from the game. Meanwhile I had the newcomer trying to get my attention. What immediately impressed me was that he pointed to his empty ring finger and asked if I was married. When I nodded NO, he gave me the high-sign and a huge smile. He had a very boyish charm when he smiled like that.

I learned his name was Wellsley. He followed me from the 55 freeway to the 91 freeway to the 57 freeway. I thought for sure that he would have given up as one freeway turned into another. Finally he motioned for me to pull over. I drove to a gas station. Cat and Mouse may seem like a foolish game, but it was safe. However, you could not be sure what would happen, once the cars were stopped. The gas station was a public place that had a lot of people in it and was very well lit, so I felt it was OK.

As he climbed out of his car, I noticed that he was very tall, around six feet at least. He was semi casually dressed, in that he wasn't in suit pants; they were more like beige dockers. I noticed he was wearing heavy gym style socks with light tan lace up shoes. His sense of style was an unique blend of avant-garde and GQ all rolled up together. Perhaps having worked amongst a lot of male gay hairdressers, I had developed an awareness about men's clothing.

When he came up to my car window, he extended his hand and offered a warm, solid, handshake. Along with the handshake came an incredibly alarming smile. His whole face enveloped his warm greeting. He could have melted an Alaskan glacier all by his smile! I told him that I was meeting a friend for drinks and he asked if he could come along. Normally I would have refused, but in a matter of seconds, I was taken in by his charm and grace. Something about him seemed so very kind. When we arrived at the restaurant my girlfriend had not shown up yet. We got to talking and the conversation flowed as if we had known each other all of our lives.

Normally when I had so little in common with a man, I'd lose interest quickly. Somehow, I found his differences very interesting. He seemed equally interested in my life. By the time my girlfriend showed up we were having an incredibly terrific time. She was pissed that I had brought a new friend along. I tried to explain that it was totally unplanned. I could not appease her and she left. Upon reflection about the sparks that were flying between us, my girlfriend probably couldn't stand the power of our connection. I couldn't have blamed her, but nor could I have stopped it….not that I had the *slightest interest* in doing that!!

Wellsley just took it all in stride. We went into the adjoining shopping mall because I needed to purchase some birthday cards. Then I needed to get back to my apartment to cook the chicken. He wanted to come along. Something inside of me said it was OK. My apartment was small but cozy. Wherever I lived, I always wanted my place to have a cozy feeling, one that people would instantly have felt "at home" in. I offered Wellsley a soda, while I prepared my kitchen. Reaching for pots and pans normally would have required me to get the step stool out of the closet. Wellsley simply reached up and brought them down to me. The joy of being tall...

I suggested that he might want to put on some music, but he declined. Wellsley was more contented to sit, watch and talk while I worked. Wellsley sat in my dining room which was right off of the kitchen. I prepared the food and we talked. Once the chicken was ready for the oven, I turned all of my attention to Wellsley.

For the next three hours we necked in my dining room. We were just like two young teens kissing and kissing but nothing more intense. I turned down his suggestion that he stay over and hold me all night. I was NOT willing to be that close with a new friend....I gave him my phone number and he said he would call me.

It took Wellsley seven weeks to call me. Before his call, I had dismissed him completely from my memory. The call lasted two hours. We agreed to meet for dinner that Friday night. It became our weekly Friday ritual for five years. For fourteen years he could light my fire!!!!

Story Four: First Date Dining

When it came down to choosing what to do on a first date, going out to eat was usually the first suggestion. I found it ironic that when women tried so hard to look good, that their dates were often not concerned at all in how they come across at the dinner table. Sometimes I wondered if it would not be helpful for all single people to be required to read *Emily Post's Rules of Etiquette* before ever going out at all. I could remember so many experiences where my dinner companion would chew his food while he talked and I had the pleasure of watching what went on inside of his mouth! The only ironic advantage to this display was that it usually curbed my appetite very quickly, and I didn't eat too many calories myself.

With all the emphasis placed on being thin, it was no wonder most single women go crazy trying to keep their weight down. I was just one of those women. Eating out was difficult because restaurants wanted their food to taste good without any thoughts about calories. If you found the dishes marked "heart-smart", those could be less fattening, but not all restaurants served them.

Choosing which style of restaurant could also be a challenge. Only in America was there an emphasis in expanding one's style of eating. All other cultures in most every other country had a more simplistic method of eating. While traveling to many other countries, I was amazed how simple the food was that the people ate. They would not ask which kind of food I wanted to eat each night. Their diets consisted of the same foods all the time. And their levels of stomach cancers, ulcers, heart disease etc. were lower than in the United States. Here in the US, it was considered boring or worse, bad taste to want to keep to one style of eating. We had a lot to learn from other cultures, particularly the Asian ones.

Personally my taste in food ran on the extremely bland side, and I wholeheartedly admitted that my style of eating created a problem in eating out. Therefore I requested that my dates not take me dining. I wanted my food to be prepared at my home. Most often my suggestion of a home-cooked meal got a positive reaction. But it was not without other problems.

I found myself wanting to put on a gourmet style meal with all the extras that went along with it. Fine china, wine (which I did not drink, but my date might have wanted too), candles, linen tablecloth and napkins, etc. The table looked terrific but did it send the wrong message?. The dinner would consist of an appetizer, main course with at least three side dishes and dessert. That came with a hefty grocery list but at least I could control the fat grams and spices. Everything had it's price....

The real problem was what happened **after** dinner. Most often, my date was then comfortable and stayed in my apartment. He wouldn't want to go out! He moved into the living room and got relaxed and talked, maybe watched TV or rented a movie for the VCR. Luckily, I did not have a fireplace. I would have been assured that laying down in front of the fire would have been a suggestion he would have made. That was not what I considered a good first date. I felt I was between a rock and hard spot. I could control the calories, fat grams, and allergic reactions to spices, or dealt with the "octopus tango" or the "horizontal mamba". (No wonder I found Latin dancing threatening).

Perhaps a new revised guide to First Dates could be created and made a requirement for all high school seniors to have read. The guidelines would be stuck in their minds for years to come. I could definitely write the chapter on Dining!

CHAPTER TWELVE

Romance and Dining

Story Five: Tripping The Night Fantastic

With all the books on the erogenous zones and where to find them, activate them, and cherish them, I had never seen one that explained how powerful the joy of dancing could be to turn two people on. Maybe there were erogenous zones in our feet, ears and hands that were triggered on the dance floor.

Obviously, the slow rhythmic "Ballroom dances" got us carried away just by watching Ginger Rogers and Fred Astaire. I never got tired of watching their old movies, even in black and white, they projected such intense romance. The "Tango" was called the dance of love, but I had personally experienced many other styles of dance, and they all had the same effect. I got so turned on by the motions, sounds and touch. After asking many of my friends, clients and even some new acquaintances, the responses were all similar. Dancing made you feel sexy. And after several hours at it, most of the people said that they were definitely turned on. But where should we draw the line? Are we just supposed to let ourselves get carried off of the dance floor into the back seat of someone's car?

When in an established relationship, going out dancing could be a form of "foreplay" for that couple, later that night. But what if you were single and went out dancing with total strangers, should foreplay be created under that scenario? I began to wonder. I had gone to so many singles dances and danced with many strangers. Some men were total gentlemen, and others seemed too eager to lay their hands upon my bottom. Then some held me against them a bit too tight while they rubbed their **lower** torso against my legs. I really wanted to scream out "hey you, when I agreed to dance with you, I did not agree to being manhandled for your own sexual release". But I never did. I just got through the musical number and made a quick dash to the ladies room while I prayed that by the time I got back, the masher was onto another unsuspecting victim. Too bad they could not be tagged when they walked in the door: *Caution, I like to rub my penis all over your legs when we dance.* Then I would have liked to stand back and watched which people lined up to dance together. That would have been an interesting "people watching experience".

I found it to be such a mystery, the balance between sexual excitement and proper etiquette… The sexual release that the music and dancing created was so pleasurable. Perhaps the men that were carried away with the sensations and couldn't have helped themselves? I wanted to be understanding. But these men were just so "groping" and felt like lechers.

On the few times that I got caught in a long musical sequence, I tried to put some space between me and my "masher", if that didn't work, than I reverted to my second plan. It was not as genteel but it got the needed result. I slipped my fingers into the nape of his neck and put a mild amount of pressure, as I softly said: "IF you didn't stop rubbing up against me, I'll be forced to inflict some serious discomfort on it." He usually didn't believe me, but as I put more tension on those very short hairs, I got the message across loud and clear. The music ended and he spent the rest of the evening as far away from me as possible......that was OK by me.

I do not want to leave the impression that going to single dances can be a real pain, because ninety-seven percent of the time, it was fantastic. You got an opportunity to get a wonderful aerobic workout, while you listened to great music, and filled your spirit with fantastic sensations. It was the sensations the body got filled with, that made it all worth while. I have gone off the dance floor and noticed that my pupils were dilated! I felt like a million dollars and wished that the feeling would never end. Alas it did. But by the time I had driven home, the feelings faded and I'd only hoped to recapture it while I dreamed.

I never knew if there was something called "Singles Luck" or something I had managed to makeup, but for many years my success in meeting interesting people at singles' parties, seemed to go in cycles. I was in one of my "positive" cycles when I decided to attend the Sadie Hawkins' dance in February. It was being held in the ballroom of the Irvine Marriott Hotel... That location seemed to bring people from all parts of Orange County, north, central and south residents did not seem to mind traveling to Irvine. The hotel was well laid out and offered many different areas to mingle and mix around. The lobby was ideally situated, if you wanted a quieter but not too cozy table for two to chat and get better acquainted.

The dance was not costumed, but a country style apparel seemed appropriate. I selected a black and gold threaded mini skirt with a form fitting white and gold satin long sleeved blouse with a sweetheart neckline and cut-out shoulders. I wore my favorite black Italian leather boots and jacket. I had my stylists curl my hair in a southern belle fashion. I even mimicked a makeup presentation that would have fit in with the look. I checked my appearance several times before making my way into the ballroom. I had no idea what would await inside. All I knew was that I was in good spirits and had high hopes for a pleasant evening….

The whole incredible experience could be best explained by telling how I met Neshda. He stood at the bar, while he watched the crowd on the dance floor. Although he was leaned up against the bar, he appeared to be about six foot. He had very thick, dark brown, wavy hair and beard. What showed of his face looked tanned or maybe he might have been from the middle east and had darkened skin. The color of his eyes were awesome, that appeared to be a white-blue color. Only in a thorough-bred husky dog had I seen such a strange colored eye. Neshda was wearing all black. From his leather jacket, shirt, trousers and boots. It reminded me of the country singer Johnny Cash. He did not resemble the singer. Neshda was an incredibly gorgeous looking man.

His body language said, leave me alone, and then I noticed his right foot. It was tapping to the beat of the music. Somewhere inside of him was the need to be on the dance floor. With a lot of hesitation, I walked over and asked him to dance. And he flatly refused. He did not attempt to make up some little white lie, but just simply said "no thanks". I was crushed, and wished I could have hid away. Just then, a man standing to the other side of Neshda, stepped up and said that he would be glad to dance with me. And we went off to dance. We were on the dance floor for several numbers, before we decided to take a soda break. As we walked back to where Neshda still stood, I tried to turn my back so that I wouldn't have had to face him. My feelings were bruised. The bartender took my soda order, and Neshda piped in "Please put that on my tab." Then I turned to him and said "I got it." Neshda smiled and I thought I would have turned to stone. I had already thought that he had the most magnificent face. I was attracted to bearded men and he had a gorgeous one, but when he smiled his face just became *knock-dead gorgeous*. He then took my left hand and kissed my knuckles. He was sorry if he appeared rude before, he said sheepishly. Then he explained that he was a very picky dancer and did not enjoy dancing with a partner that could not follow. I watched you and Gill (the other man-who turned out to be his room-mate) out on the floor, I knew I had misjudged you." Nesda said with strong confidence. I decided he was either the most arrogant man I had met in a while or just outlandishly honest. But that smile had given me tingles and so I decided to stay and talked with the both of them. Gill decided to take a hike, and I felt a bit odd about that, I had not meant to make him feel like the third wheel. Later I learned that he and Neshda did this double evaluation a lot. I was not sure why, but then I had never figured out why men did what they did most of the time…

He removed his jacket and his shirt fit him like a glove. Although I could not see the muscles underneath, it was apparent that he was very well built. Neshda took me to the dance floor. I had watched Astaire and Rogers a zillion times, and dreamed that I miraculously turned into Ginger Rogers. For the first time in my life, I actually felt like Ginger! I was amazed as I caught my reflection in the mirrored walls. It was almost too fantastic to be believed. People on the floor gave Neshda and I more room to dance. He dipped and twirled me like a true master. Now I understood why he was so picky about his partners. He took his dancing very seriously and wanted a partner that allowed him to do what he wanted. Until that very moment, I would never have believed I could be maneuvered the way Neshda orchestrated. It was almost unbe-lievable. The second time I caught my own reflection, I knew I hadn't dreamt it. I was in seventh heaven. IF only the Deejay would play a long set. I did not want it to end. When the music finally stopped, I was float-ing on air. A crowd had formed and when we stopped, they applauded. I was embarrassed and pleased all at the same time. I looked up at Neshda and said: "Thank you for making a long standing dream come true. I had wished to be Ginger Rogers for eon's and tonight you made that happen. I am truly honored, thanks." I started to walk away. I assumed that he would have wanted to dance with others. I was content with the one glorious night of dancing I just had. He called after me: "Off to the bathroom?" He wanted me to come back to the bar when I was through. I could not have believed my ears. This was going to be a great night!!!!

I pretended to dash off in the direction of the rest rooms, and then walked just as briskly back to where he stood. I had a sixth sense that by the time I got back, there would be a line of women waiting to get onto the dance floor with Neshda. After all, we had created quite a crowd of on-lookers. And I was so right, they encircled him two layers deep. There must have been ten or eleven of them, all different ages, sizes and appearances. One tall, willowy, blonde was rubbing up against his shoulder. Although it would have been worth it to "wait in line", my own ego couldn't allow me. I turned quietly on my heels and made my way to the front of the bar. The Deejay started to play "Lady In Red", my most favorite song. I had a jab of regret that I had not forced my way to Neshda's side. I focused my attention to the dance floor, watching the pairs as they made their way to enjoy the melodic rhythm. When I felt my hand being slid into someone's palm. The second I looked up my heart skipped a beat; it was Neshda. He said this was his favorite song and should only be shared with me. If I had died and gone to heaven, I could not have been more thrilled!! We danced all night long. I usually left these dances early, but not that night. We were the very last ones out the door.

I had not believed in love at first sight. I had never experienced such delight in all of my life. The magnanimousness of it was beyond words. Never before had I ever considered letting anyone follow me home. IF Neshda had asked, I thought I might have said yes. But he was a complete gentleman.

We got together the very next day. It turned out we were both writers and he was in need of a professional editor for a technical manual he had created. My sister Jackie would have laughed out loud had she heard when he made such a request. Jackie was my editor of all of my work, and knew that I did not have any talent for it. Regardless, I immediately volunteered to help him.

I barely got to sleep that night. I was so excited with the idea that we would be working together. I wanted to make a great impression. In the forgiving light of the dance, anyone looked better. Now we were to work in broad day light and all my insecurities came rushing into my head. I couldn't decide what to wear, how my hair should be styled, plus my makeup too. So many decisions and so little time....I decided on my favorite David Hayes red and black wool suit with a matching silk blouse. I wore my hair down and chose light pastel makeup colors. Except for red lipstick. I wanted my mouth to appear sexy and kissable. We had not been at all romantic with each at the dance. Normally I wished for men to be more gentlemanly, however, Neshda had driven me crazy and I had wished and dreamed how it would be to be kissed with his beard against my skin. Would his kiss be tender to demanding and rough? So far I hadn't a clue.

Initially, it was supposed to be a quick one-hour review. To do the job correctly, took four weeks. During the editing, we had to meet many times. Sometimes for lunch, at a local restaurant. Each time I struggled with my appearance. I was so taken with his, and so far he kept an arms length from me and did not approach me in any manner that could have been mistaken as sexual. Than I offered to make dinners at my condo. Neshda changed his approach towards me on the second dinner. Since it was at my own home, I dressed in a casual white satin jumpsuit. I wore no jewelry, no underwear, and only a trace of makeup...Neshda took me in his arms upon his arrival and kissed me for what seemed a blissful eternity. Only the fire alarm going off because the chicken dinner was burning, caused us to separate. I wasn't hungry for food anyway. We ordered take-out and laid on the floor in the livingroom, 10% worked on his manual and 90% spent on kissing. Without a doubt Neshda was the finest kisser I had ever met in my life. Sensations that he caused with is lips and tongue are beyond description. I would if I could, but I tried and failed when I wrote letters to my closest friend. On the third dinner, we ate by candle light. If it was not love, I did not know what people called it. We never consummated our love. Whether Neshda knew something about the future that I had no clue of, or for other reasons that I also never understood, it simply did not happen.

Neshda left for Paris, for personal reasons. I gave him a dozen postage paid postcards pre-addressed to me. I got a few and then not a word. I would always remember our special nights. And that fact that he had made my dreams come true. On the first night I truly was Ginger Rogers, and Neshda was my Fred Astaire. All the others were just as special and I had no regrets....

Story Six: Dancing Without A Shroud Of Smoke

Sometimes it was easily understood why people who were married got jealous of those of us that were single. From an outside observation, being single provided a freedom and a sense of adventure that ended once you were in a committed relationship.

One such event was a singles smoke-free dance that was held three out of four weekends. I had attended the organization's parties for over ten years. Although months and months had gone by between my visits, I counted on meeting some very interesting and often times very different kind of people. One of the reasons the group's attendance was so high could be contributed to the variety of locations that were chosen to hold the events. Many came from backgrounds, and "walks-of-life" that I had never experienced. These people were so fascinating to me. Perhaps I seemed unique to them too.

The smoke-free dance was held on the Friday night that started the four-day Labor Day Weekend. The head organizer had selected a wonderful restaurant over looking the ocean. The balcony alone was the perfect romantic setting for any couple. Four-day holidays could be a real bummer for singles. Without a significant partner to plan some interesting outings, single people were left to find events to fill the long weekends. The long Labor Day weekend was one of those holidays…so I went to the dance. With the location being such a terrific one, I felt certain that the turn out would be positive. The goal was to enjoy the evening with at least one fascinating person.

As with all singles events, presentation did play a large role. Therefore, I spent extra time selecting my outfit. I was probably like many women, who would go through their entire wardrobe and swear that they had nothing to wear! Finally I had chosen a favorite of mine, a red jumpsuit with teeny white poke-a-dots that had a plunging low-cut back and sweetheart neckline. It couldn't have made me appear tall, but it did make me look thin! One out of two wasn't bad. With my hair flowing down my back, the deep plunging back didn't look too revealing. I wanted to look sexy, but not like a slut. With precision that twenty years provided, I made up my eyes as only a professional makeup artists could. I was pleased with my reflection and drove to the restaurant feeling jubilant.

Once inside, I was seated at a table along side of the dance floor. I sipped my soda and watched the people as they walked in. I adored "people watching" and these dances provided endless opportunities to do so. That particular evening I was wearing a small cap that matched the color of my jumpsuit. It went well with my outfit and my high spirited mood. As Mischa walked along the outer corridor, he caught my eye and gave me a smile that I registered as one you gave someone you thought you recognized. My memory was like a colander, information went in and left pretty quickly. Therefore, he might have met me before, and I had no recollection. Not wanting to let on that I hadn't recognized him, I returned his open smile with one of my own. As he came over, I could not place him! He came over and told me that my hat suited me well. Then he added a comment about me being one of the most striking women in the room. I blushed and immediate understood that was a pickup line, albeit a good one. And I was relieved that I would not have to maintain the charade of recognition. Clearly I was a stranger to him too! Then he asked if he could sit down. It was a good thing I attempted to say yes, because he had moved next to me in less than a second.

As I mentioned before, I was seeking to meet fascinating people. Mischa (pronounced Me-sha) was one such person. Mischa was aggressive, that was apparent. Aggressiveness was a real plus in my book, as long as it was not mixed with arrogance and or inappropriate behavior. I quickly learned that he was a probation officer. Similar to police officers, it was a job requirement to be assertive. He applied these skills to his social encounters too.

Mischa was six foot two, with a strong masculine build, and gorgeous teeth. When he smiled, his face changed dramatically. His physical strength was heightened by the powerful impact of his smile. He definitely was charismatic! Along with his strong sense of self, came a great flare for dressing. Mischa was wearing an Armani grey suit, and light salmon colored shirt with a white collar. He had cuff-links of black onyx and gold with a nugget watch and pinkie ring. I had no idea what a parole officer made, but he looked like a million dollars!

Then we went onto the dance floor. I learned so much from being in a man's arms while dancing. The first few numbers were fast melodies and I was not impressed with how he moved to the rhythm of the music. Just as I decided that I needed to get back to my table and watch some more, the Deejay put a slow number on. With the grace of a gazelle, he swept me into his arms and moved around the floor like a real pro. I must have had a look of surprise on my face, because he whispered into my ear: "I was born to slow dance, I need to feel my partner's body against mine to get into the music." And boy did he ever! Not the disgusting pelvic thrusting some jerks forced on you, but real smooth, wonderfully powerful and tremendously thrilling maneuvers. I would have never gotten off of the dance floor except that the style of music went back to rock and roll. Mischa simply guided me back to my table when the music changed. Next came the uncertain part, would he make a graceful exit or sat down again to chat.

Not wanting to make him feel that I was monopolizing all of his time, I waited to see what his next move would be. He went to get a drink from the bar, as he departed he said: "I'll be right back." Often used as an easy exit line, I decided to resume my people watching. The fact that he hadn't asked if I wanted a fresher drink, I took that as a sign that he would be gone. I simply smiled and looked away as he went off to the bar or whatever…

Seconds later, another man plopped himself down on the chair Mischa had just given up. On looks alone, I would have been in trouble. The man wore two opposing plaids on his shirt and pants. The colors were not even the same, although both had red, blue, yellow and green in them. His hair appeared to be coated with a full tube of VO5 hairdressing oil. It was almost so shiny that I could have seen my reflection in it. Had I stood up, we would have been about the same height. "Hi, doll, I saw the other loser leave such a dish like yourself" he retorted. Like that was supposed to impress me? Then he said that I could now have the pleasure of a "real guy". He extended his sweaty hand with chewed up fingernails. We all had name tags on, so I said: "Please excuse me BOB, but my brother just went to the bar and would be back shortly." I knew I was lying but without being openly rude to him, I wanted him to take a hike too. It also allowed me to "save face" if he hadn't returned. Luck was in my corner that night. Mischa walked back my way while Bob hadn't left. I flashed him a look of "**HELP**" and he did just that....He walked up to Bob and said: "Excuse me that's my seat and it would be appreciated if you got lost!" Mischa smiled at me and added for the effect: "Hi honey sorry it took me so long the line was longer then I expected." Bob was all of five feet four inches in shoes, and he sized up the situation and skidaddled. I was very grateful that Mischa assisted me so well. But I was embarrassed, because I did not know what to do next.

As luck would have it, he solved that problem and asked me to dance. "Lady In Red" was playing and it was my all time favorite slow dancing song. It felt so good to be in Mischa's arms. Particularly when I could dance with someone that did it so well. He looked down at me, since even in high heels I am only five foot four, and said "Boy we certainly have some kind of chemistry." I wondered whether I had spoken my thoughts **out loud** by mistake! Embarrassed I just nodded in agreement. I was hoping for a long set of slow numbers, I only got part of my wish, we danced for two more. By the time the set was over, I could have floated on air.

To recapture my sanity, I excused myself and went to throw some cold water on my face. When I returned, another woman was seated on my chair. Now my chair had my coat on the back, a drink in front of it, along with my driving gloves. Except for a blind person, you had to know the chair was spoken for. I slowly approached my things, not sure what I should do. I decided to give up my perfect table, since Mischa had helped me out earlier, I did want to appear grateful. Just as I picked up my coat, he asked if I was leaving? "No" I said. I thought three's a crowd and I would find another spot. Mischa then introduced me to the **very** lovely-looking, tall, blonde female. His co-worker was named

Marsha. He explained that they were in the same district and had just learned that information a moment earlier. Then he turned to Marsha and told her I was his new dancing partner. I introduced myself as "Miraeh."

"Miraeh was my nickname and I used it when I attended singles events. It protected my need for privacy, from the "*Bob's*" of the world. By the way Mischa introduced me, I could tell that he did not want me to leave. And so I put my coat back and stood next to Mischa. He offered me his chair but I declined. As far as positioning goes, standing with shoulders touching was more the kind of message I wanted to send to Marsha. She had other ideas. The conversation preceded to cover work related topics. And so I just stood and listened, and listened and listened. I was almost ready to give into to her plan, when the song "I only have eyes for you" was played. Marsha was in mid sentence when Mischa stood up and said "It's our song," and took my hand as he got up from the chair.

I was so very surprised and pleased at the same time. On pure instinct, I just kissed him smack on the lips and said "Oh you remembered!" Something in my head wanted to go along with the ruse. While on the dance floor Mischa apologized for the situation with Marsha. And then he kissed me, and I mean really kissed me. The chemistry on the dance floor was nothing like the sparks I got by his kiss. I was not someone that condoned such sexual expression in public. But it was really terrific. By the time we got back to Marsha, we were arm in arm. She finally got up and left us to our own communication.

Funny thing about meeting strangers, if there was chemistry between you, it does not seem quite as important to have a lot in common. Without chemistry it would be the major determinant if you would continue to speak at all. With Mischa, it was clear early on, that our interests were not in sync, but it did not stop us. We spent the rest of the time together. I always left these parties early and this was no exception.

As I left, he asked what I was doing the next night. "I planned to walk around the Orange Circle." I replied.

For the last thirty years, the Circle of Orange has had a Labor Day Celebration that brought over one million people to attend. "Would you mind company?" he asked. We agreed to meet there at five thirty, after I closed my salon.

I was a bit nervous about meeting him. Did my hair and makeup look OK?, Had I looked fat in my outfit? The lighting at the dance was far more forgiving than broad daylight. Of course I had one of my stylists do my hair that afternoon. I went for the sides to be pulled up and most of it cascading downward. I had brought five outfits to the salon and had the entire staff critique them all. We all selected a blue and white slacks outfit that had a darling red and blue short blazer jacket that went over it. I looked festive without looking costume-like. I was able to wear my brand new LA Gear sneakers without ruining the look. I needed comfortable shoes for all the walking we would be doing. Mischa saw me first and by the look on his face, I could put aside my self doubts. Again he was dressed to the nines. He had on Italian pleaded white trousers, and a light blue shirt with a white v-necked, cable knit sweater. He also had white sneakers on. His eyes were even more sparkly in the sunlight. I was certain that my face must have registered how attracted I was to him. He just smiled at me and I tingled from my head to my toes.

There was so much to see and do, we spent hours working our way through the crowd. Around nine thirty p.m., he said that he had to leave. I was disappointed but tried not to show it. That was far earlier than a normal Saturday night date would end. He made plans to meet me at my home on Monday morning for another date. The date ended with several wonderful kisses and hugs.

Sunday afternoon I got a call from Mischa. He canceled our date for Monday. I was so surprised. But what he told me spoke **volumes** about the dating world! What I was not privileged to know was that *after* I had left the dance, Marsha and Mischa had taken back up with each other. That meant that he had spent from six p.m. to ten p.m. with me and from ten-fifteen to two am. with Marsha. Then on Saturday, when he left me at nine thirty, it was because he had a date with Marsha at nine. He had been a half an hour late for that date. His date with Marsha ended with a stay-over on Sunday and all that day too. He thought that he had found someone he was going to "take up with". I wished them both good luck. I took his business card and threw it away.

I would miss having such a fabulous dancing partner. He would never be a Neshda, but with Neshda living in parts unknown, the Mischa's of the single world would have done quite nicely.

Story Seven: Funny Things Happened On The Way....

The Mischa story had a second part, that followed the first part, three months later. The Christmas season was rapidly approaching. That was one holiday that was not any fun alone. Being single forced me to go out to another singles dance in the hope that I would meet an interesting man. Obviously my goal was then to start dating. IF luck was looking my way, I would then have had the opportunity to have an escort for some upcoming parties.

With that agenda in mind, I got ready in my usual fashion. The selected outfit was a silver and gold dress and jacket. The organizer had selected a very posh five-star hotel as the location for the smoke-free dance. She was the same person that had organized the dance that I went to over the Labor Day weekend. I had not attended any other dances since then. Putting one of these events together was no small feat. The smoke-free dances were put by a woman named Mitzi. She should get a medal for all of her hard work.

I arrived early as usual to get my "preferred" seating. It worked like a charm. Within minutes a gentleman walked up to me and asked if he could join me. His name tag read "Don", mine said "Miraeh". Don took my hand into his and kissed my knuckles. I would have wanted to laugh, except his accent reflected an European background. And his silvery hair indicated that he was of the generation that would have been trained to greet a woman in that manner. Somehow the gesture fit him. Personally I was tickled to death. I asked him where he had been born and was told "Bulgaria". I hadn't a clue where that was exactly and didn't want to show my ignorance by saying so. I hoped that he wouldn't ask me something in reference to his homeland. Luck was in my favor because he went on to say that he moved away at the age of eleven and hadn't ever returned. He added something about it being so different now with all the wars and political strife in the region. Even though Don had left his homeland as a young boy, he still had an accent. Men with accents seemed sexier somehow. His made me think he might be from a Baltic country. Don was dressed in a very conservative manner with tweed trousers and a white shirt and bow-tie.

Although men age more subtlety than most women, it was apparent that Don was several years older than me. It didn't bother me at all. I found him an interesting person to talk to. Mischa saw me talking to Don and walked right up and interrupted our conversation with "I saw you on TV talking about your book," as he gave me a wink and a dazzling smile. That was a total lie and we both knew it. I wanted not to embarrass him. I replied: "It aired at 6:30 am. Sunday morning, boy you must have been up early." I turned to Don and explained that I had written a few books and one very small show called *Main Floor* had interviewed me.

That was not a lie. The taping was done in Florida the year before, and my segment had aired then. *Main Floor* did air on Sunday mornings at six thirty am. So it could have happened as Mischa implied.

Mischa wanted to talk to me but I was not willing to end my conversation with Don. I told Mischa I would catch him later and he took the hint and left. Although I wasn't willing to stop speaking with Don, I couldn't have helped noticing how gorgeously dressed Mischa was that evening. He wore another Armante suit only this one was navy and tan. He wore a tan shirt with a matching tie and whatever they would call the "hankie" that sits inside of the small breast pocket of the suit coat. Even Mischa's shoes matched his suit. Boy oh boy could that man dress!!!! An hour later, when I still hadn't ended my chat, he came back and interrupted with "Hope you don't mind but that's our song". "Lady In Red" was on the Deejay's system. This time I agreed and got up and danced with him. We still had that chemistry on the floor. He leaned down and whispered that he had looked for me at several dances. He wondered where I had been? I replied: "You could have called me at home if you needed to reach me so badly." I refused to give into the chemistry.

"Did you and Marsha come here?" I asked with sarcasm in my voice. It always seemed strange that single couples would show up at a singles dance together. Singles that went to these socials attempted to meet someone. So when you have someone in your life, how logical was it to go where everyone was open to hit on anyone else???? Mischa shook his head and rolled his eyes as he tried to explain that he had hooked up with another "*Fatal Attraction*". She turned out to be **nuts,** he cried, and drove him crazy. When he realized he wasn't getting any sympathy from me, he tried to turn our chatter back to finding out where I had been all these months.

He repeated how he had looked for me at several of these dances, and was surprised I was nowhere to be found. Mischa than told me that he had run into one of my girlfriends at these dancers, many times. And each time he asked about me. I was not the least bit impressed with his attempt at being forlorn about not seeing me for a while. First off, the woman he mentioned was anything but a friend, and secondly, ı not really his business where I had spent my time. Softening my thoughts, I told him that I never attended all the dances. In fact wh had met him months earlier, it had been over a year between soci. Besides, I had been very busy with my career.

Mischa then tried to pull me into his chest and whispered: "You coul\ have called me." I just shook my head and laughed. With an air of indif ference, I explained that after the last phone call, I took his business card and threw it in the trash. Quite frankly until he walked up to me and Don, I hadn't given him a second thought, much less desired to call him. The song ended and I went back to my seat, Don was still there. I spent the rest of the evening with Don.

The very next morning I got a call on my personal line, it was Mischa. He wanted to try to be friends. Something told me "friends" was not what he really had in mind. Casual sex was not up for consideration, for me. Chemistry was indeed rare and could be quite terrific, but it was not the only ingredient that made for a good lover relationship. The Mischa's of the single world had not learned that yet!

Story Eight: The Girls Club

I never understood why women went to clubs in packs. I went alone. Once I walked in, the whole room was filled with other single people, so what was so difficult? Watching the women all around me, I noticed a pattern that made being approached so tough. If I could see it, why couldn't they?

Whoever said men were the stronger sex, had never watched one as he walked over to one of these "female packs". He had to deal with several pairs of eyes watching his approach, and then continued to watch as he selected one woman and asked her dance. If the woman turned him down, he was forced to handle all of their rejected eyes. The whole process was tough enough that it challenged the most confident male. These women should have taken the initiative and broken up in pairs. Then the man would have had an easier time as he made his approach.

From my twenty years of experience, these women were usually very attractive. I was not saying that they all would have made the **cover** of a glamour magazine. However, they usually wore a good deal of makeup, coiffured hair styles, and their dress sizes were all under size ten. These women were in-touch with what was currently in fashion, and their wardrobes reflected the *rave* of the month. When seated in their *pack formation* they either giggled or talked a bit louder than was necessary. They wanted everyone else to notice them.

Many times these female packs showed up at the same singles bars or clubs every weekend. They actually began to take over "territories" which meant that they were seated in the same spot every week. If unsuspected newcomers sat in these chairs, wow, look out, there would be *trouble*! I had even seen a group of women that forced the newcomers out of their seats! Just once, I would have loved to see the newcomers refused to move and instead suggested that the "pack" found other arrangements. I could have wished for it, but it never would have happened.

Women, that are heavier than thirty pounds over their ideal weight, sat by themselves. Somehow they knew they needed to make it easier for the men to approach them. Sadly, since most men were so visually stimulated, the heavier women had a more difficult time to compete with the willowy stick fingers of the "girls club".

Sometimes I pondered what would have happened if all singles events were conducted in blind-folds. Then the sound of the voices, the way their skin felt, the silkiness of their hair, how they smelled, what they had to say, would all have made stronger impacts than what they looked like. At the end of the evening, they could have removed their blinders and seen how they looked... hopefully their impressions throughout the evening would hold more credence than what their eyes registered. Unless of course they ended up really looking like perfect Ken and Barbie Dolls! With the popularity of the TV show: *America's Funniest Home Videos*, I have wondered what would be the result of secret tapes from one of the local "hang-outs" one weekend night. Then to have been able to witness what their reactions would be to the tapes as they were played back on the wide screen TVs in the bar….it just might have been good enough to have won the ten thousand dollar prize. I was certain some would not have found themselves funny, but maybe they would have learned something that would have changed their behavior.

CHAPTER THIRTEEN

Creative Ways To
Meet Mr. Right?

Story Nine: Before There Were 900 #'s

It was late Spring, around the last week in May, a Thursday evening, around 10:00 p.m. and the telephone rang. Although it was not too late for me to have received a call, I had not expected one. So the phone startled me a bit. I had been relaxing in my living room, reading a romance novel by Judith Michael. I had been all wrapped up in my favorite silk-threaded afghan. I jumped up from the cozy stuffed rocking chair to catch it before the answering machine got it on the fourth ring. Just as the fourth ring was just about to peal I had the receiver in my hand. A tiny bit out of breath, I attempted to sound soft, and sexy as I said: "Hello". Since I was single, I could only hope a late night call might be from Wellsley. I heard a deep, sexy baritone voice reply: "Hi baby, tell me what you're wearing this very moment?" I was immediately disappointed. He obviously had the wrong number, and must have misdialed his girlfriend's number.

I knew when I was in a hurry it happened to me. I felt a bit embarrassed, as if I had accidentally intruded on what was meant to be a private moment. I became flustered. I wanted to let him know that he had the dialed wrong. I couldn't help being drawn to the sound of his voice. I replied: "You have gotten a wrong number, please don't be embarrassed. Have a nice night." I put the phone back in the cradle and went back to my cozy living room chair. I returned to the book and wrapped myself up in the warmth and serenity of the afghan. In less than five minutes the phone rang again. This time I was sure it must have been Wellsley. So I answered with a sexy, "Hello". The male voice said: "Hi". It was so short a reply, I just assumed it was Wellsley. I continued with "Evening sweetheart, you'd never guess what a wrong number I just had, while waiting for you to call." In my ear I heard a deep, soft, sexy laugh. I immediately realized *I* had been *mistaken* and asked who it was? He said: "Why your sweetheart of course", as a bit of laughter still rang in the undertone of his words.

Now I was embarrassed and mad at being made fun of, when I had just made an innocent mistake. The caller sensed my dismay and tried to calm me down with using his deep, rich, baritone voice, and spoke softly: "Don't be upset, I was so taken by your concern with my misdialing, I decided to call back to tell you so." I recovered quickly. "Oh that's OK, I have misdialed many friend's numbers when I'm hurried." He asked: "Do you like to talk on the phone?" I told him I loved the phone, my friends thought I was crazy for my attraction to it. I then added: "I could talk for endless amounts of time". My friends knew that if they needed to speak to someone even very late at night, that I would have always taken their calls." I was not sure why I felt it was OK to reveal so much about myself. Looking back on it I would see that I was more than a bit foolish.

Thinking that this should be about the end of the call, I started to say "Good night." I was taken by his next response. He said he was not in a hurry, at all. In fact, he had all night. He still wanted me to tell him what I was wearing right then. "Excuse me!" I tersely replied. I had not liked the question. He was not taken back by my tone of voice. According to him, we had just met under unusual circumstances, and that he found my voice very beautiful. That made him curious, and tried to picture what the rest of me looked like." Somehow it sounded logical, although upon reflection I would surely see it differently.

I was willing to admit to myself that I had put my "voice" on. It was the sexy tone I tried to use when speaking with Wellsley. And I had to agree that when I do, I knew that others have commented on what a change it made on the phone. Ever since I was a small girl, I developed a special "phone voice" that I could turn on and off quite easily. My mother used to say it was very beguiling. So perhaps I had caused this stranger to inquire what I was wearing to get a better idea with whom he was speaking. I only had a blanket wrapped around me. I always wanted to reduce the amount of laundry anyway I could. Re-dressing to stay alone in my apartment just never seemed "laundry-saving".

Obviously, I could not have told that stranger that information!! Instead I quickly remembered what I had worn to work and began to describe that outfit. I finally replied: "I have on a red and blue blazer, with matching blue trousers and white blouse." His answer annoyed and insulted me. "You decided to get ready for the Fourth of July parade six months early!?" He was laughing while he said it which only further added to the feeling I was being insulted. "*Well excuse me*, are **you** some fashion critic?" I retorted angrily. I liked the appearance of the liberty colors, and the outfit looked good on me. I felt that he had made me defensive. He noticed my sarcasm this time and decided to change his tune. He tried to explain that he hadn't meant anything bad by that, he guessed because it was late evening by most people's standards, I might have been in some silky nightgown. Before I knew what I was saying, I blurted out "I don't wear anything to bed." Immediately I wished I had not said it. I was even more embarrassed that he knew something so personal. I could not take it back and tried to switch the conversation in another direction. Unfortunately, he was very interested in that declaration. If he sensed my embarrassment, he had not let on. Instead he offered the following: He also slept naked, it was so much more comfortable to have slept without the confinement of pajamas. He felt that if more people just realized that, the lingerie business would be in big trouble. Then he added how he admired a sensible woman that knew what so many others hadn't found out. I was not sure whether he was just trying to placate me or if he really did mean those words. Regardless, it made me feel better.

Then he began to ask some other probing questions. I was to tell him the length of my hair. He wanted to know if it was silky, straight or curly? What color were my eyes and shape of my lips? Why these questions didn't set off an alarm inside of my head, I couldn't say. Maybe the sound of his voice had enchanted me so, that I was willing to go along just to keep the conversation going. Regardless, I did answer his questions. "I have slightly wavy, auburn hair that ends in the middle of my back." And it might have felt silky, I took extra care of it, I told him. My eyes were very dark brown, I called them cows' eyes. People said they were my best facial feature. My bottom lip was a bit fuller than my top and I had that natural bow on my top lip.

He commented "What an unusual way to describe yourself? Descriptive on one hand, but not sensuously. I expected you to play along better than that?" I was taken back as if slapped on the wrist like a child. "I did not realize that this was a game, and that there were rules to follow", I snapped. "I think it best that we end this call, your apology for the first call is accepted" and hung up. And did by letting the phone drop into the cradle with more of a bang than I had really intended. However, I was mad and felt that if it had caused his ears to ache, so much the better. We had not even exchanged names, and when I looked at the clock, I was shocked to see that I had been on the phone with this stranger for more than thirty-three minutes. That was a long time for a wrong number!!

Four days would go by before the phone would ring again with the golden voiced stranger at the other end. If I was honest with myself, I would have admitted that on the following night of the first call, I kind of waited to see if the phone would ring around ten. No call came that night. Then I put it out of my mind. When the phone rang, I didn't have any thought of whom might be at the other end. The second I heard his voice, I was surprised how it effected me. Why my reaction was so strong, escaped my logic. None the less, I wanted to try again and hopefully have a better result than the last call. All of the sudden I felt tongue-tied. I simply did not know how to proceed. He must have felt the same, because he was not saying anything either. I started to tell him if he had not dialed my number by mistake we should have introduced ourselves? My name was …"and just at that moment he interrupted me with a demonstrative "NO DON'T!…please let my fantasy linger on a bit longer. Let's make up names that best described what we thought of when the other was speaking. He continued with his reason for calling me Mariah. "Like the wind you were soft, but powerful, your voice could be gentle as a breeze that tickled my ear or rough as a storm that beat my temples senseless." I was shocked NOT by his request, but by the way he was so poetic. I had not heard anyone speak quite so eloquently and I was really impressed. I even loved the name he had chosen. In fact it was one that I had often liked in books I read. I meekly agreed and then began to ponder what I might call him. Bronson came to mind. So I replied: "OK , I shall call you Bronson". Because it sounded like a stylish man, with unusual tastes. He laughed and said: "Fair enough Mariah, Bronson it shall be." He wanted to know how I was that evening. Had he caught me in a patriotic mood, or was I being more sensible to enjoy the freedom in being nude?

I was glad that he could not see how red my cheeks had become. I was indeed comfortable in the privacy of my living room with just socks on. I recovered quickly and said: "I actually have my favorite pair of grey argyle socks on, and no I am NOT ready for bed just yet. I like to read a romance novel, before starting my own dreams." It made me sleep better and I had more enjoyable dreams that way. Bronson offered "What a clever girl you are, to help your subconscious mind with words of others. Have you ever tried to create your own fantasies, without the assistance of another writer?" I was not sure if he had attempted to voice his disapproval of my reading selection, or just had offered an opinion. I felt uncomfortable about speaking about fantasies. This might not have been a good idea after all.

As if he sensed my hesitation to continue, Bronson decided to share with me what he was wearing. In a deep, melodious voice he spoke to me. "Mariah, I am standing before you in only a satin, black, thong and a huge"…then paused and let my imagination wonder, and continued "smile just hearing your voice. Now tell me again what you are wearing?"

"Sorry Bronson," I said. "I was not comfortable with this game." "If I had said anything before that gave you the impression that I was, please forgive me." I thought this was a good time to say goodbye. I sort of expected him to chaste me or call me a baby. I would have felt compelled to simply hang up, if he had done just that. However, his tone of voice became very soft and gentle. He apologized for bringing me into a game that he liked to do and thought that I would be opened to it too. Then he made the zaniest suggestion. He asked me if I would critique a story he had written. I asked what the story was about, just in case he would have begun to read to me some weird or kinky porno material. I did not come right out and ask if it was pornographic literature. My hesitation was very noticeable. My voice had an edge to it that I had not used before. I had to give Bronson credit when deserved. He did pick up on my uncomfortable feelings and said: "Mariah, I could read this story to my mother. So do not worry about the type of content. He said nothing more that gave away the plot or story line. He wanted me to decide for myself what he had written. Bronson was interested in how it sounded to me. "Are you ready?" he inquired.

I said I was. He suggested that I got comfortable and turned the lights down low, and lowered my stereo. I had my favorite opera Puccini on and I did not think he could have heard it. The volume knob was on one, so I turned it off... He then suggested that I lit a candle, and relaxed as he began reading. Bronson turned his voice into a deeper, richer, more velvety tone and started:

> It was raining so hard against the windows that a melodic rhythm could be heard. Charlotte loved the rain and if she were spending the evening alone, would have loved to build a fire, open a bottle of her favorite white zinfandel wine, and listen to classical jazz on her CD player. Instead she went running around the cabin picking up the strewn papers and books getting the place presentable for Jacque. This was to be their first dinner together and she was very nervous. Charlotte wanted everything to go well. First she would have to pull off pretending to be a good cook. The Italian restaurant on the corner was family owned and not a lot of people knew it. All of their dishes were homemade and so when she explained her dilemma to Mamma Lionnei, it was decided what dishes would be prepared and all Charlotte had to do was bring Mamma her very own casserole containers and it would look like it came from Charlotte's own oven. The complete dinner cost her a weeks pay, but if it went well it would be worth the expense. Next the candles were set all around the place. She looked at the clock, and decided it was more important that she got her bath, hair and makeup done than spend more time cleaning up. As she walked

into her bathroom, she looked back into the main living area and wanted to kick herself for not being a better housekeeper.

Charlotte had been to Jacques many times and knew what a great place he had. At his apartment, everything was perfect inside. She had put off this event for as long as possible but the day of reckoning was here and she made the best of it. After going through every outfit she had in her closet and her best friend's too. She was lucky that her best friend's clothes were her same size. The navy velvet dress was selected. It was short without being a mini, the velvet nape was still rich looking even though it was six years old. And she could wear her diamond pendent and earrings. She wore her hair down and soft curls since she used Hanna's electric curlers. And with the help from her facialist, she had gotten a few tips that made her eyes look more sensuous. Just a drop of gloss over her lips and she was ready.

Jacque was punctual as usual. He devoured Charlotte with his eyes. A bouquet of roses were held behind his back and with his free arm, he pulled her towards him and gave her a long, French kiss. Charlotte found herself being pressed harder and harder into his body. They would have stayed in the doorway a lot longer but a gust of wind blew her dress up to her waist. Jacque hadn't noticed. His eyes had not left her face. Charlotte pulled away from the embrace and invited him in. She suggested that he should make himself comfortable. She then walked into the kitchen to see to the dinner. Casually over her shoulder she told Jacque that the wine was on the coffee table. He poured them both a glass of wine. When she returned with the appetizers and plates, she was quite surprised at what she saw. Jacque was laid prone on the couch, and had taken off all of his clothes. She couldn't hide her shock! "You said to make myself comfortable didn't you?" he said as he saw her expression. And of course she had, but hadn't realized this was what he had in mind. Not really knowing what to do, she just put the food and plates down and sat on the couch next to him. "Let me help you get more relaxed" Jacque said as he unzipped her dress in one smooth motion. He must have been very good at this, for she hadn't been able to get the zipper to work that fast when she was dressing. In seconds, she felt his hands as they slid the dress off of her shoulders, down around her waist and would have gotten it to the floor if she hadn't been sitting on her bottom. No sooner than that thought was in her mind, Jacque pulled her on top of him and slide the dress off. All the while he was kissing her neck and the edge of her shoulder. Then he slid his tongue inside of her lacy bra and had her nipple in his mouth. As he suckled her breast, she could feel the hot heat rise from inside of her thighs. Charlotte did not feel the release of her bra or her panties, but she could feel how tingly his fingers made her as they explored all of her body. When he placed his fingers inside of her, she thought she would go crazy with delight. She cried out in pleasure. While their bodies united, he whispered "Now it felt like I was home."

There was a long pause on the phone. I did not know what to say. This was not a story that I would have read to **my** mother. But having Bronson read it aloud as he had, it did sound wonderful. I felt like it was a tender story and very personal. Perhaps from Bronson's own experiences. So I asked: "Where did you get the material from, was this autobiographical?" Bronson laughed and said "Did it matter?" No not particularly, I was just curious. But regardless it was very good. "Are you planning to do a complete book or just short stories?" I asked. Once again Bronson sensed my confusion and explained that it depended a lot on me. I was still confused and did not know how I made a difference. "You see I felt inspired when I first called you and felt that I had met someone that could provide me with the motivation to continue my writing." he said with a plea in his voice. I could tell he was trying to coax me into agreeing to help in his work. This was why he has asked me what I had been wearing that evening. He said he had hoped to create new material for his book. "Won't you help a fellow writer?" he pleaded again. I should have declined and let the whole incident end right there. But at that specific moment, it sounded like a legitimate request and one that would not take too much time. Soon I would learn how wrong I was.

Bronson ended up calling three times a week, always late at night and he always wanted to speak of sexual feelings, and intimate experiences. For the first week it was kind of fun and I had never experienced "phone sex" before. Bronson was very imaginative, and most of the things he talked about, were new to me. Admittedly, I had not been a promiscuous teenager nor was one as an adult. Some of his shenanigans ended up helping me with Wellsley. I was able to suggest an idea or two to Wellsley after I had heard from Bronson. Wellsley always seemed pleasantly surprised. After careful consideration, I decided it was not a good idea to tell him where my inspirations were coming. But the calls did have their negative side too.

By the third week it got boring. And by the fourth week I changed my phone number. Since he never knew my real name, my privacy was saved. However if I ever heard a strange male voice on the other end of the phone ask me "What was I wearing right then?…." I would just hang up.

Story Ten: Blind-dating At The Melon Stand

It has been said that you can meet your next Prince Charming at the grocery store. It was not supposed matter if it were a large chain or a some small independent store. The idea was that you could learn a lot about a person from their shopping cart and have had a lot to converse about while in the store. There must be a lot of single women out there believing that was true, because lately I had noticed so many well dressed women, with great hair and makeup presentations, shopping in the produce departments. But for the life of me I didn't see any flirting that went on. The few men in the store, at the time I noticed these women, were not paying any attention to them.

Then in September, one Wednesday early evening, I had finished my last client early and decided to do some much needed food shopping. There was a "Von's" in the center where I worked. Before leaving my facial room, I removed my lab coat, checked my hair and reapplied my blusher and lipstick. Just in case I were to run into a "client", I would have looked presentable....yeah right! I could fool some of the people some of the time, but I too was just making sure I looked OK for the "potential" unexpected encounter....

I was not in a particular rush to leave the store. That was a rare occurrence in itself. When I noticed a young college aged woman trying to make conversation in the lettuce section. I could tell by the way she kept tossing her hair and batting her eyes at the cute grocery clerk, that she wanted him to notice her. From my position, which was much too far away, it appeared that they could be about the same age. He was around six foot, short, blonde, crew-cut styled hair. His store uniform did nothing to show off his physique, but his arms seemed to imply that he worked out faithfully. I definitely understood her attraction. If I have found a version of him twenty years older, I would have been batting my eye lashes at him too. I could not resist my curiosity and wheeled my way to the bananas to get a better view, and perhaps to able to have overheard a word or two. Just as I got my cart in place, I heard him say he did not know the differences in the lettuces. He suggested that she check with the produce manager. He had just started working in the store that day. I tried to hide my amusement, after all she did not need to know that someone else witnessed her rejection. Maybe rejection was too harsh an interpretation, perhaps he hadn't picked up on her flirtation signals. He didn't show any real interest. I was sure she wasn't too happy about it.

However, just as I moved my cart and got away from the scene, I bumped into another cart over at the melons. A man had also been intrigued by the lettuce incident and had watched not only the two college students, but my reaction and interest as well. Talk about being embarrassed. Now the shoe was on the other foot and pinched everyone of my toes quite nicely!! I blushed a few shades deeper than my already cosmetically prepared face. I tried to make a quick get away. But alas I failed. If I hadn't been so embarrassed I would have been able to notice how good he looked. The stranger was also tall, approximately six foot four. He had salt and pepper hair, with more "pepper" than salt. His eyes were a blue-green, which seemed to match the pull-over sweater he had on.

He stopped my cart by putting his hand out and said, "It would be a shame if the moment slipped by without at least two people saying hello." He had a slight brogue sound to his words. I couldn't have placed his accent, although I found it appealing to listen to. He told me his name was Gerald and asked what was mine. I meekly replied "Shelley". "Was that with two E's or one?" he asked. My attention immediately was drawn to the fact that he knew the difference, and had not asked if it was a nickname. Even most of my relatives sent cards addressed to Shelly. It's the way most people thought to have spelt it, except for my mother. The name Shelley was the nickname for so many other good names: Michelle, Rochelle, or Sheldon.

Gerald had a great smile, his eyes crinkled when he did. He also had fantastic looking teeth. If I could have afforded any kind of cosmetic improvements, my teeth would all be capped. His looked real though. Once he smiled, my embarrassment waned. Quickly we began moving around the store together. I had brought my normal list not because I was so forgetful, but it kept me on a tight budget. Which I definitely needed to follow. I would be very prone to impulse buying IF I hadn't kept to a list. Gerald had a different method. He did his shopping while the alphabet ran in his head. As he went down the letters he would remember what he needed. I was amazed on how that worked. I asked "Doesn't that make you go back and forth the same isles a lot?" He replied: "If I was in a new store, it would." Otherwise he just kept the letters in his head as he walked down the isles. He was able to remember which letters were to be found in which part of the store." Then he told me that shopping was not something he liked to do or did often. He took his time and expected to spend two hours in the store. By the time I had finished my list, he was only a third of the way through his process.

I enjoyed myself immensely, but needed to get home or my frozen foods would be soggy. I extended my hand to say goodbye, when he asked if he could have called me. I gave him my business card and began to turn away, when he called after me. I rolled my cart backwards when I heard him say: "Was there a man at your home that you needed me to call you at the office?" Startled, I said: "No". I owned my own business and was just more comfortable when I gave out my business number rather than my private number. We had just met and this was easier for me. I was at work more often than at home anyway, and it would have reduced the chance of "telephone tag."

His next comment really was the shocker. "Well my wife would mind my getting calls from a gorgeous woman". So he never gave out his home number either. He was not wearing a wedding ring. There were no female products in his cart, no baby food, ice cream bars, sugar cereals, or pampers. These were items that would have indicated the status of the home front. I just about reached over and took my card out of his hand, when I changed my mind and told him that I never accepted calls from married men unless they made appointments for facials. It sounded like his wife deserved a special treat of pampering. I suggested that he consider one of my gift certificates for her. "Have a nice day." I said as I walked briskly to the cashier. That experience lead me to give up the search for "Mr. Right" at the grocery store!!!

Story Eleven: Puppy Love

I was not sure when one would be too old to have experienced puppy love. Before I walked into the bookstore and literally ran into Ken, I thought it was considered a term to describe two very young children who found out that there was a difference between girls and boys. In elementary school, puppy love hit around five to six years old. Or even in Junior high, we got huge crushes on fellow classmates.

On the evening of June 10th , I was late for a party and needed to pick up a present. There was a great bookstore called "Bookstar" nearby my salon. I could get in and out very quickly. That added to my decision to find a present there. I had rushed to change into my silk, purple jump-suit as my last customer was paying her bill. I had quickly pulled my hair into a modified French twist. An hour earlier I had redone my makeup. Therefore getting a present was the last item left for me to do. I would not have walked into a party empty handed. I did not know the guest of honor very well and thought a book would have been a good choice. Upon reflection, it probably was one of the more difficult choices I made. What made me think I knew what she would like to read? Maybe it was just fate that took its course so that I would be able to see Ken again.

Wow, Ken was some man! There he stood, five feet seven inches, thin build, with light brown curly hair and pale blue eyes. He was wearing a

Baltimore Orioles' baseball shirt and tight blue jeans with Nike tennis shoes. Not much different in appearance then when I last saw him in Junior High. He did not have the mustache of course, but his height and weight were similar to what I remembered. Ken had managed to keep his youthful figure. Maybe it's a woman thing that makes us so easy to spread out. Even his hair hadn't looked as if it had thinned out too much.

We had been in the same homeroom in seventh grade, English Lit, and our lunch breaks were together. By the time we were in the ninth grade, I had written "Mrs. Shelley (Ken) in every loose leaf notebook I owned. Besides my diary entries, my best friend, Ilene knew how much in-love I was with Ken. Unfortunately, Ken thought of me as his best pal. We talked about everything. Well almost everything. He had such a crush on Brandi. I thought she was a stuck up bitch. Ken thought she was the prettiest girl in the school. Looking back on it, he probably was right about her appearance, and I was correct about her personality. Regardless, I remembered reading in the newspaper that they had gotten married after high school. Back then, I had ripped the announcement out of the paper and burned it. That was fifteen years ago. Time healed old wounds and gave a lot of perspective to the situation.

I was in a hurry and crossed over one isle to the paperback book section of the store when I smacked right into his shoulder. It took a second to re-compose myself and I began to say "I was so sorry", even before I got a chance to see who I just plowed over. I started to stammer…. Oh, my G-d, was that Ken??!!!. I could hardly believe I had been so clumsy, let alone that I had managed to come face to face with my past. It seemed to take a moment for him to realize that he knew me. So I said: "It's me, Shelley from Sudbrook Jr. High." He smiled while he rubbed his shoulder and laughed, "Well I'll be….boy it has been such a long time, I'm surprised you knew who I was?". "Actually you have not changed much besides your mustache.", I said. He grimaced and replied that he certainly hoped so. Ken added: "I was pretty gangly in school, and I've filled out a lot since then." He looked terrific to me and I said so. What brought you out here to the West Coast?" I inquired. We both grew up in Baltimore. "It's a long story," Ken said, as he looked at his watch. I took that as a sign that he was in a rush. I had actually forgotten why I was in the book store, and then add I had to be going too. "I was on my way to a party and needed to get a present." I tried to explain why I had been such a clutz. I wanted to have the chance to speak some more, so I suggested we could talk over coffee some time? We both seemed to want to bring each other up to date with our current lives. Ken agreed he would like to get together but he would be flying home the next day. I realized that I had only one chance to make this opportunity work. If he had the time, he could accompany me to this party. I would make an appearance and then we could go for a drive and talk. I hoped he would agree but I really could not make out from his body language what went on in his mind. I began to worry that I came on too strong, when he said if I thought it would be OK to crash the party, he would have loved to spend some time with me.

We spent fifteen minutes at the party. Nobody would have really cared much if I had not shown up at all. Ken and I headed for Laguna Beach. I was never much for playing in the sand and surf. This area had so much to do and see, that it was the perfect place to chat and be relaxed. We could have just walked through all the art studios and found something that kept the conversation from lagging into uncomfortable silence. Since it was his first trip to the Coast, he allowed me to pick out the areas of interest. I selected the downtown strip with all the quaint shops and galleries. As it turned out, we had no problem with things to say.

Brandi turned out to be a living nightmare for Ken, and after ten grueling years, they divorced. It left him emotionally battered and had not seriously sought out anyone to date ever since. They had one son, but Hal had turned against him ever since the divorce. It seemed that

Brandi had made Ken out to be the rotten one in the whole matter. I just listened. I had learned that it always took two to make or break up a relationship. But decided it was best to be quiet and let Ken tell it his way. Meanwhile he had changed his career several different times. One of the key problems Brandi and Ken had was over money. According to Ken, Brandi did not think that he ever made enough. This was why he was brought out to the West Coast. His new employer had sent him on a training course for new product knowledge. I asked what the products were and he just mumbled something about conduits and conductors. I decided his lack of enthusiasm and the sound of what I thought it might be about, it was better to leave it alone. Next I asked about his family and how he was feeling. His family were about the same. I always forgot how things on the East Coast stayed the same when here in California change was embraced by so many people. In fact I thrived on change. Ken turned the tables and asked me about myself. I told him that I was still very single, loved my work in Holistic health and had published five books with three more coming in the next few years.

Unlike Ken, my physical appearance had changed a lot since Jr. High. I had always been very heavy as a child, and if he had seen me three years earlier, I would have appeared obese. But I was eighty-eight pounds thinner, and my hair was auburn in color and very long. When I was growing up I had always had very short pixie style hair cuts. I had let my hair down from the French twist I had worn earlier. I just ran my fingers through my hair and let it cascade down my back. I had hoped it didn't look too bad. He must had read my mind because he glanced down at my hair and said: "I should have grown my hair long back in school". Ken had always liked long hair on women. In fact it was Brandi's long hair that attracted him to her so many years ago. Boy if I had **only** known, I would have grown my hair longer than Rupunzel's!!

I decided I did not have much to lose after so many years, so I said: "Ken you probably would not remember that I had such a terrible crush on you all through Junior High and most of High school too." Ken blushed and then without any warning, took me into his arms and kissed me. At first, I was too shocked to respond exactly. But it did not take me long to return his kiss. We stood there on the Laguna Beach pier, and kissed for what seemed an eternity. Finally, Ken broke away and softly said: "Isn't it ironic that the most wonderful things we had right under our own noses we took for granted?" I just smiled and curled under his arm as we walked back to my Mazda GLC.

"Are you hungry?" I asked. He responded: "Not right now". We headed back to my condo in Anaheim Hills. If we got hungry we could whip something up there. "If my memory served me right," he chuckled " you were always the domesticated one of your family." He wondered if I still liked to make people dinners. I laughed. I had forgotten how long ago my interest in the culinary arts had started. I had thought that to be a perfect wife you had to know how to cook, bake, sew, knit and darn...and so I learned them all!

We got back to my condo, just as the sun set. I was so grateful that I was one of those "A personality" style housekeepers. I didn't have to worry about the place being a mess, it just never was....My condo was three stories and had three bedrooms and three bathrooms. I was comfortable in it, although it was big for just one person. My furniture was eclectic, each room had it's own motif. The second floor was all done in southwestern colors. The living room had two matching woven textured ivory, sea foam, and sienna colored couches and two sienna and teal big stuffed chairs. The carpeting was new and I had chosen a cream colored Berber. I had one of those gas powered fireplaces, and one paper log ready to be used. Ken attended to the fire as I went into the kitchen and found us some munchies. By the time I had gotten back to the living room, Ken had the fire going, my candles around the room all lit, and my Barbra Streisand's "Memories" played on the stereo. I was glad that he had made the room so cozy, and that it seemed natural for him to do it.

I brought two glasses, his with wine and mine with soda. I said "Here's my favorite toast: May we live for as long as we want, and may we never want for as long as we live." Ken than gave his " Here's to old friends finding each other and beginning again." His eyes registered the question: Had I thought we could? I just nodded since I did not want to lie but was not sure it was possible. We talked and danced in the living room for hours. I couldn't believe it was one thirty in the morning and I wasn't a bit tired. Ken felt the effects of the wine, and the three hour time change from east coast to the west.

We walked arm in arm upstairs to my bedroom. My room wasn't too feminine. He commented on how much he liked the king size, brass canopy bed. My satin comforter was black, white and rose colored. My sheets and king-sized pillows were black satin. We ended up making love all night long. In the morning I got up a few minutes early and prepared the roman bathtub for us to share a luxurious Aromatherapy bubble bath. Much to my pleasure, he had never had one before. We made love again, as if it would have been our last. The passion and intensity was almost too much to handle. There were no words to express our inner feelings and turmoil, so we just held each other tight and said nothing.

I took him back to his hotel and stayed with him until his plane took off at LAX. We made no promises that couldn't be kept. We agreed to write and to call as often as we could. In the first month of his return to Baltimore, we spoke almost every night. As the weeks passed, we got more caught up more in our own lives. The calls were less frequent, and the letters were more informational, than words of love and emotion. After three months, it was apparent that Puppy Love was a wonderful memory but not something to grow on.

I would always remember Ken as my first true love. My memories kept him in a special place in my heart forever.

Story Twelve: You Never Know What You Will Find Right At "Home"

Richmond was six foot tall, with black hair, blue eyes, smooth deep olive complexion and perfect pearl-white teeth. We met in a peculiar way. We both lived in the same apartment complex. It was gigantic, with one thousand, eight hundred units. I had lived in my two bedroom/ two bath apartment for five years. I knew less than a dozen people by name and maybe twenty-four more by general appearance. It was a warm day in December, and he had washed his red, Ford pick-up truck in the area that ran along side the entrance to my garage space. Normally he would have used the car wash area for his building but management had tarred the roof, so no one was allowed to walk there. I had just done a large grocery shopping run. In keeping with my motto, "you never know who you'll run into in the store", I had on a snug fitting teal jumpsuit. It had a great belt that accentuated my small waist. Although my backside was always larger than I would have liked, I was currently on the slimmer side of my sliding scale. Like many other women, I was perpetually gaining and losing weight. At that time, I was down about thirty pounds, which always made me happy to celebrate......

I was having a party that weekend and needed a lot of supplies, paper goods, beverages, and all the ingredients for a lot of homemade Jewish dishes. I was preoccupied with making several trips from the car to the apartment and carried several bags of groceries each time.

Although I was oblivious to it, he had watched my behind as I made my trips back and forth. I told him that a true gentlemen would have offered to help me. His defense was that I should have asked for assistance if I had needed it. Oh the troubles the women's movement had created for me. Some arguments were not worth pursuing. We both agreed to have different point of views. Now back to how we met....

On my last trip, he was finished with cleaning his truck. He called over to me and said: "Did I have a huge family or was I having a party?" I laughed and said "the latter" and continued up the staircase. Richmond quickly followed. It made me nervous to hear his footsteps so close behind me. I panicked and wanted to be able to go anywhere other than my actual apartment. Then I spotted an older female neighbor at the end of the short hallway. I did not personally know her, but I knew she had lived there many years before I had moved in, and that she was about sixty years old. The woman's apartment door was opened as if she too, was expecting someone. She had on a faded pink sweatsuit and barefeet. Her hair was all grey and not combed. I couldn't tell if she had just awakened or was about to go to bed early.

Since I was in a pinch, I decided to walk towards her. I was not sure what I would say when I reached her doorway. So I waved hello as I got closer to her. I thought I was safe from him following me, when Richmond stopped there too. He said: "I didn't know you were friends with Carolyn?" I was baffled and didn't know how to respond. Just then Carolyn broke the silence and said: "I thought she was with you Rich, what could we do for you miss?" It turned out that Carolyn and Richmond were platonic roommates. All I could do was to invite them both to my party. Richmond immediately accepted, Carolyn gracefully declined.

He then followed me back to my apartment and we chatted while I prepared my menu and arranged my kitchen for all the cooking I needed to do for the party. I made chopped liver pate, baked a brisket for mini sandwiches, whipped up four different kinds of blintzes and created two kugels, one sweet for a dessert and one loaded with cheeses for my vegetarian guests. The process took hours. I told Richmond he could leave at any time. He seemed contented to stay and watched me work. While I cooked he looked around my place and commented on my artwork and my style of decorating. Although he wasn't forthright in his opinions, his facial expressions lead me to believe he was very much impressed with what he had seen. My tastes ran on the ultra modern motif. Almost everything in the apartment blended in the almond lacquer and gold theme. All the furniture was streamlined with smooth edges. The art on the walls and the statutes in the entertainment center were from contemporary artists. If nothing else could be said of my living quarters, it was neat and tidy.

Richmond had not been exposed to Jewish cuisine before, so the smells that filled the air were different for him. He was *very* curious, and asked so many questions I could not keep up. I did my best and answered most of them. Finally, I told him he was free to taste what he wanted, and leave anything that didn't appeal to him. Richmond laughed heartily. He loved new experiences he retorted with a wicked twinkle in his eye. Somehow I felt he had suggested more than the experience of new foods.

Once he was in my apartment, and I no longer felt my security was being threatened, I really took a long look at him. He was *extremely* attractive. I decided to play along with his banter, "What exactly constituted a new experience?" I asked and winked. He smiled and I felt my heart skip a beat. I knew I began to blush. I got nervous as I felt his eyes roamed all over my body. Richmond complimented me by calling me a very fine looking woman. He questioned why we had never met before? Had I just moved in, he wondered?. He shared Carolyn's apartment for a year, and was certain that he would have remembered if he had seen me before. I had a hard time adjusting to being asked so many questions all at once. "No", I replied, "I have lived here for more than five years". I tried to turn the situation back to him so I mentioned that I hadn't ever seen him either. I attempted to return his strong gaze but was not as comfortable with it as he seemed. Richmond had been seated on one of the breakfast nook stools. He then got up and put his arms around me, and in a throaty voice suggested that we got properly acquainted. With that comment said, he pulled me towards him and kissed me. At that moment I knew I had a new neighbor that a simple nod or smile would not suffice, as I walked down the hall.

Richmond must have had similar thoughts. He explained that before that afternoon, he had tried to stay away from the apartment except to sleep, shower, shave and sh—t. He had many different reasons why that had been the prior arrangement. That afternoon changed all that, he would be glad to come home from now on. Richmond's expression showed how happy he was. I did not want to crush his excitement, however it was a bit more than what I had in mind. I was very touched by his openness.

There were tremendous differences in our backgrounds, and lifestyles. Plus I was many years older. I had never before had a friend, male or female, that was eight years my junior. If anything, I tended to date men, where I was ten years younger then them. My last relationship was with a man fifteen years older. Being the one who was older made me feel uncomfortable. Richmond tried for three years, but I never got over it.

The time I spent with him was totally unique and we were always excited to see each other. Only in the quiet moments in my room, when everything was dark and my mind re-canted various experiences of my life, did I ever re-think whether I had made the right decision. No matter how I reviewed it, I still came up with the same conclusion. I would have never traded the opportunities we had shared, but I was certain that we were not meant to be together as a couple.

We are however, still close friends. We talked on the phone several times a year. We sent each other cards for our birthdays and holidays. A few of our experiences were so memorable that I was compelled to include them in this journal.

Story Fourteen: When Do You KNOW That You Have Met "Mr./Miss Right"?

When we began to date in high school, our parents encouraged us to play the field and date several different people. In our twenties, it was still thought to be an effective dating process. Many parents would have said: "Go out with many men/women to make sure that you have "sewed your wild oats" so that you would then be ready to settle down to have a family." Even with the divorce rate raising past the fifty percent mark, men and women still planned to start their families shortly after college. Waiting until after you reached your early thirties to have a family was not looked upon as a viable goal. If more had waited, perhaps the single parent rate would not have risen so high.

As we matured, a different pattern to dating developed. Men and women alike, felt compelled to stay "off of the market" at all costs. We would have gone out with someone, and if the first date was acceptable to both parties, the idea of dating exclusively became understood. The second date was often set up before the first date was over. Because the idea of being "on the market" was so loathing for most people, the desire to connect was paramount. The process continued as long as both people were willing to do so. I had heard from friends and clients that they were willing to continue to date a person even IF they did not exactly enjoy their partner, just so that they did not have to go back to being "on the market" again.

Which brought me to my own dilemma. I had never forced myself to do the above. Therefore, I had found myself in a lot of first and second dates without seeking to accept the third offer. After ending a fourteen year relationship, I was faced for the first time to decide what I wanted to do with myself......being "on-the-market" did not appeal to me either.

Recently, I had met Ned. He was close to my own age, was of the same faith, and had a brilliant, creative mind. Physically Ned was very cute, he had soft curly brown hair, light green eyes and a full beard. Although somehow the hair of his beard was course and gruff. But I figured with a good hair conditioner, it could have been turned into a smoother sensation. He had perfect looking teeth and a smile to melt an igloo. Ned was tall around 5' 11", very thin and not very muscular. I hoped that meant that he was not going to be a devoted jock. In addition, he had many qualities that I admired and respected in a person. Since I had not known him very long, I could not say with complete certainty that he was honest and trustworthy.

There was an aura about him that felt good, this was a special quality that I found enormously appealing. In addition, I adored facial hair on men, along with hairy chests. He had both.

So far he sounded terrific! And I was thrilled to be able to say so. There were two elements to Ned that had caused me some concern. First, he was separated for only six months. If I agreed to continue to see Ned, I would be the "re-bound" relationship. That would put me at great emotional risk. I could have gotten emotionally attached and then had to deal with his leaving to try to make the marriage work....

Second was that his behavior could be considered immature. Since I had just met him, I was not sure that I could call it that. It was very possible that he was just in touch with his *inner child*. So often we were forced to remove ourselves from our past jovial behavior. I would not have called that immature behavior. The two may have appeared on the surface to be the same, but the latter allowed us to use poor judgment under certain circumstances. The former allowed the freedom to react to situations like a child would. It was too early to determine what Ned's behavior should be considered.

Case in point:

Yesterday we got together to go to lunch at a wonderful café called "Crocodile Café" and then to the movie "*Mar's Attacks*". He was so eager to see it, so I agreed to go to a movie that I had zero interest. At lunch he played with his food as a young child would do. Then he blew bubbles in his iced tea with the straw. During the movie he played thumb wrestling with me. Again I just went along with it. That was our third date in less than two weeks. A good sign that we might have started a pattern there.

We got back to my apartment, we settled in the living room to chat and cuddle. To passionately snuggle at the very start of any relationship was a tough call for me. For the thousands of women that went to bed on the very first date, that would NOT have been a concern. Then there were those that followed my pattern, where intimacy went slowly. It took me a long time to feel that it was the right time. Cuddling was one of those "border-line" kind of physical contacts. It could have been just a way to express affection, and started the process of getting comfortable with each other. Or it could be interpreted as a form of "foreplay". The former was what I had in mind. But was that what Ned thought? It was also not easy to ask for clarity before I began…at least I had not found a way to do that. Instead I just began with light massage movements as we talked. My fingers stayed on his shoulders and the back of his neck. Being a licensed masseuse, that came naturally to me. The holding and kissing was also very nice. Luckily for me, Ned did not take our cuddling as a signal for sex.

Even though the time spent was so very pleasant, there was a child-like quality to his manner. I enjoyed being with Ned. Our dates lasted over seven hours, and the time just flew by. That was unusual. Since I had so much experience in dating, I knew that a normal date lasted about five hours if it went well and three and half when it didn't. However the baby-like quality to his behavior had caused me some distress. That evening he brought it up in conversation. "Was I immature?" he asked of me. Now I was taken completely by surprise. I believed that the truth should be told. However, total honesty could be devastating. I tried to be honest and politically correct at the same time. Well I was not sure, actually, I offered timidly. He must have realized that I had just begun to get to know him. I went on and said that he was probably a man that got in touch with his *inner child*. Had he thought he was immature, I asked? He giggled liked a small boy, tilted his head to one side and said "I dunno ." The subject was dropped. But I could not get it out of my head.

Long after he left, I re-played our dates in my mind. So much of the time had been terrific. The inner child/immaturity issue did bother me. Nobody's perfect, so maybe it was best to let it rest and continued on as we had been......I did look forward to seeing him again. I hoped he would call soon. I was not liberated enough to have made the first call. I would gladly have returned a call but could not get enough nerve to have initiated it. Helen Gurly Brown would NOT be pleased with me.

Story Fifteen: It is seven hundred and twenty hours and counting....

If you were married would you ever have wondered what it would be like to be in a twelve year relationship as heart-felt as a marriage but without the legal document? Or if you were in such a relationship, had you given any thought to the process that you'd have gone through if it had ended? I never did, that was until the day it happened. For the first time, I was forced to realize how lonely the process might be. I had no idea how much frustration would occur as I attempted to become single again. For the first few months after the split-up, I endured tremendous confusion and isolation. I just didn't fit into a comfortable social niche.

With marriages, you were given a period of time to separate before the relationship dissolved. Lawyers got involved and the process took about one year. In that time you had the opportunity to deal with your thoughts about what was important in your life and your partners'. Although the dialogue between the two of you could have gotten heated and ugly, the chance to discuss things would have come up a lot.

But what about a relationship where there was no legal document called a marriage license? These relationships could have been just as emotionally intense. You would have begun each day with one another and end the day the same way. Your partner was probably the first person you went to and told all the specific details of your every day events. When you do not have children, the communication could have stayed focused on the two of you. That was how it was with Wellsley. Look at the background. We had known each other for fourteen years. Twelve of those we shared every aspect of our lives with each other. Most days began by talking over the phone if we had not slept together the night before. All nights ended with speaking either directly or on the phone. Throughout the day, we were in constant contact. It was not unusual for us to have called each other five or six times a day. The phone company loved us. We loved each other.

No subject was too mundane, no topic too sensitive to discuss. There were so many parts to our relationship that were important, we were best friends, and family to each other too. Both of our families lived out of state. His were on the west coast (Washington), mine were on the east coast, Virginia and Florida. Neither of us could have easily "popped over" to visit on a weekend. Everyone wanted to keep in closer touch, but it was always difficult. Large phone bills took the place of plane rides. Each of our relatives thought of us as a couple.

We had no boundaries….except for one. After ten years, I wanted to take the relationship to the next level…to actually have gotten married.

Wellsley did not. I felt that I needed more commitment in the relation-ship. Signs started to appear slowly that made me wonder if Wellsley was still feeling that he was in a committed relationship with me. I had reasons to suspect that Wellsley was "roaming" into other women's bedrooms. My work required me to do a lot of traveling. And although that would have provided me the same access to waver from my com-mitment to him, I was never tempted. The old clichés began to have new meaning: "Out of sight, out of mind," and "While the cat's away, the mouse shall play." Under a marriage contract, that was clearly understood, and, legally, would not be permitted. Although I had felt that we had similar guidelines, it became apparent that I was very much mistaken.

Since the legal issue of fidelity did not exist, all of my other friends felt that I should have expected him to cheat. That simply hadn't made a lot of sense to me and I had a lot of time to think about it, b-e-l-i-e-v-e me! I was surprised about how little support there was for those of us that were going through the process. There were no group meetings to go to either. I had seriously considered starting one....

Fourteen years in total and I had to make the toughest decision of my life. I either needed to be connected with someone else who was partial to the idea of marriage with fidelity, or I could have stayed with the lim-itations Wellsley set forth.

With heart wrenching clarity, I decided to move on. (Ergo I met Ned.) Not a second went by that I was not thinking of Wellsley. A song on the radio, a TV show or commercial, a movie plot, or billboard sign would have brought to mind a memory about our lives together. Everywhere I went, I couldn't escape from my past and my heart. Could I successfully win this battle? Only time would tell...but if you are a betting person, place your chips on "YES". After all, it has already been seven hundred and twenty four hours as of yesterday, and counting...... And I have made another date with Ned for the weekend.

Story Sixteen: A Wolf in Sheep's Clothing

Once you have reached your fortieth birthday as a single person, you are automatically tagged as being too particular. This title was one that I especially hated and felt was most undeserved. Here is a prime example of why I held that opinion.

It was Spring and the weather was gorgeous, a time in which a woman's thoughts turn to the idea of sharing her life with a significant other. Such was the case with me. Since the facial salon business is not ideal for meeting eligible bachelors, I turned to my tried and true social encounters...i.e., a single's dance. I found one listed in the local paper and I got myself all psyched up for it. The location was in a great club called "Music City," known for its do-op fifty's motif and music. The whole club would be used by the group, so no smoking would be allowed. That was an important element because of my life-threatening reaction to smoke. California's generous no smoking polices were greatly appreciated by me and everyone else that suffered from the same severe allergic reaction to cigarettes, cigars and pipe tobaccos. The music would bring out the older single population of Orange County. Fifty's style songs had not made a big hit with the 30-something crowd but for forty and over, it provided nostalgic memories. Going onto the dance floor would flood my head with terrific thoughts of my past.

My weight was on the lower side of the scale, which prompted me to wear a short, purple silk dress. I had inquired earlier and outfits from the past were not requested. Purple was a color that made me feel good, and silk is a marvelous fabric to wear while dancing. Then I selected the right accessories, and I drove myself to the dance. Once inside, the small talk and banter began. Alas I was seated at a table right off of the dance floor. That made it less threatening for to a man to have approached me. By making my location ideally situated, anyone could have come up to my table, or politely moved on and no one would have been the wiser. As I have already pointed out, the process of rejection made it tough on the man. Because I was so aware of that, I never refused a request for a dance. It would not have killed me to dance at least one dance, no matter who asked me. Believe me I have had my share of two-lead feet stomping all over my toes, my bottom pinched, my breast tweaked, and various other unfitting onslaughts. And yet I continued the process.

When I spoke to other friends and or relatives, they simply had not appreciated the effort that was made, just for the chance to connect with a really nice person. After all, if I was there, and I considered myself a decent human being, surely there were others just like me at the same dance. That was what I continually told myself as I prepared to go to these events.

That evening I met Ben. Early in the evening he approached my table and asked if he could sit down. I smiled and accepted his invitation to join me, realizing that there was some risk involved. Having a total stranger share my table could have put me in a compromising situation. If we didn't get along, it would become awkward. First, I would have to give subtle hints, hoping that he would then pick himself up and leave. If being subtle proved ineffective, I would have to decide what to do next. One option was just to make the best of it, knowing that no other men would approach me the rest of the night. A second choice would be to leave the table myself and relocate. I always hoped that I did not have to make that choice. As in business, the key to success was: Location, Location, Location! That could be applied to a single's event too.

Luck was in my favor, Ben was very charming. He was fairly tall, five foot eleven inches. His suit was attractive and showed that he took very good care of himself. His salt and pepper hair was wavy and shiny. It appeared that he had just gotten a haircut. That always tipped me off to the level of interest a man had with his appearance.

A man should care what he looks like in public, particularly since it does matter to most women. I realize that women are known to fuss with their appearance a lot more, but that should not dissuade men from taking some time with theirs. Two areas of interest to me are the teeth and hands. If a man has well groomed nails, it says he cares about himself. Ben had hands that showed good care.

Besides nice looking hands, it's just as impressive to have great looking teeth. When a man smiles and you see beautiful clean teeth, it makes such a good impression. Ben looked perfect when he smiled as he approached my table.

One other minor detail that really makes me take notice is if the man wears old-fashioned cuff-links on his shirts. That is one men's accessory that has never lost its power to make positive impression. On that evening, Ben had black onyx and gold cuff-links on a pale blue Italian style shirt. His collar was custom-designed with very tiny embroidered initials on the edge. He wore grey linen pleated trousers with suspenders instead of a belt. In my opinion, he was a very dapper dresser. As he approached me, Ben looked fabulous. First impressions are very powerful. No one ever gets a second chance to make one.

Although I spent a good deal of time noticing his appearance, it wasn't the most important part of his presentation. Looks were just part of the package and I was a woman who felt that on an overall judgment, looks were **not** the most important! The more important first impression was yet to come. It depended on what Ben would say. Could he hold an intelligent conversation? I was not sure, but eager to find out.

At these dances, I wore a name tag that did not reveal my real name. An event in my past led me to do so. I used my nickname and spelled it in an uncommon way. "Miraeh" is used to convey "Mariah". I loved to watch people's reactions. Some showed an immediate discomfort with a name they had not seen or heard before. Others tried to determine my ethnicity by it and proceded to jump to a variety of wrong conclusions. All of that always amused me. Ben just walked up to me, extended his hand and said; "I don't believe I have ever seen a name like yours. How do you pronounce it?" I smiled and was inspired by his direct take-charge manner. I replied: "Ma—rye—a." I explained that it was a nickname, chosen by my friends because they said that I was very talkative. And, just like the wind, I could be a powerful force to be reckoned with. I matched his firm handshake with my own. Oh, how I hated a "wet-noodle" handshake. Ben's was full of confidence and I liked that a lot.

We danced most of the evening. By the end of the night, I was very glad that I had made the effort to go out. Ben asked for my number and I gave him my home number. That was not the norm. Most often I just gave out my salon number. But, after spending most of the evening with him, I decided he was really a nice man. He asked when was the best time to reach me, and I explained that very early morning or late at night were best. When we parted, Ben suggested that we should get together soon. I went home very happy.

When a week went by without a single message from Ben, I decided that I had been mistaken after all. And I wished I had stuck to my old pattern of giving out my work number. Oh well, what was done was done. In the middle of the next week I got a call from Ben around midnight. The hour did not alarm me, but he did sound a tiny bit intoxicated. I was not certain, though, as I could not remember his voice at first. Our conversation was brief; he wanted to know if I would like to go to the movies that Saturday night.

Once again I must refer to all of those so-called friends of mine that kept telling me that I was too selective. My own opinion was that a movie on the first date was a terrible choice. It shows NO imagination, and no attempt to interact with the person. I kept all of that to myself and simply agreed to go. I did not even mention that thrillers and gory flicks really bothered me. I told him that I was finished at the salon around five-thirty and we agreed to get together at six-thirty. I really wanted to meet him at the theater, but he insisted on picking me up. Again I did not resist. Instead I gave him directions and said good night.

Saturday afternoon arrived and I realized that no mention of dinner had been made. I had not wanted to assume that we would have dinner together, so I ate a very late lunch. Just my luck, my last appointment at the salon canceled and I got home a half hour earlier than planned. I took a quick shower, re-touched my hair, and changed into a black jumpsuit. My outfit would fall into the category called: nice casual. I remembered how well Ben was dressed the first time I met him. I decided that was a good choice. It was ten after six and I was ready. I never agreed with the idea that you should keep your dates waiting. If you agree to a time, you should be ready when they arrive. Now arriving time was where the story got interesting.

By eight o'clock I had not heard from him. I went through my usual bouts of worry that something might have happened and anger that Ben had not called. When ten p.m. came around I got ready for bed.

The following weekend I attended a lecture on being single in the nineties. Maybe I would learn something about the dating process that I had not known before. If nothing else, everyone there would be single too. And low and behold, who sauntered in?....good ol' Ben! He was wearing the same great outfit he wore the first time I met him. He came right over to me with a big broad smile, and expected an equally warm greeting from me. Not so! My eyes were full of distrust and a bit of annoyance. Time settled me down quickly, so he didn't receive the wrath I would have been able to offer. Ben was puzzled by my cold reaction. I simply stated: " I am not interested in speaking to any man who stands me up. Please excuse me." And I began to walk away when he reached across and grabbed my arm firmly. "What had I meant by being stood up," he asked with a look of confusion across his face. To his knowledge, he had not done anything of the sort. That infuriated me. I let him have it in a very low but stern voice!! Ben's face registered shock and disbelief. "I honestly have no recollection of any of that" he cried. He must have tied one too many on when he called me. He seemed genuinely sorry. But had no memory of ever speaking to me, much less making a date. He pleaded with me to allow him to make it up to me. I remembered that I had thought he sounded slightly intoxicated, and so I decided to let it pass. Once again we spent the evening listening to the speaker and chatting during the break. By the end of the night, we agreed to go out to dinner and a movie the very next evening. I knew he was NOT drunk when he asked that night. Once again he insisted on picking me up, so I gave him my address and directions. He was to come over at seven p.m. I even teased him as I left, that he better be early this time!

I went through the normal ritual of getting ready for a date. I selected a peach dress and matching sweater. Movie houses are often cold inside and I wanted to be prepared. When the phone rang at six fifty-five. It was Ben saying he was running late and would be there at seven thirty. Quickly he got off of the phone. I hadn't been able to ask whether the change in time would mean that we would not be able to go to the movie or perhaps change our dinner plans to a light snack after the show. Then it dawned on me that I didn't know what movie we were supposed to be going to, or what restaurant he had in mind. In addition, I noticed that he had not seemed a bit apologetic about the change in timing. I decided to dismiss it all so that we could have a nice evening once he arrived. I was ready early as usual. To pass the time, I watched some local news. When the clock on the screen said seven forty five, I began to wonder what was up. When there was a knock at my door at ten minutes to eight, I was already fit to be tied. Timeliness is one of my pet peeves. Ben just walked in and said, "Well, we missed our reservations." He wanted to know where would I suggest we go that did not require one. I had not known where we were going in the first place, so I did not know what to offer as another choice. Even if I still WANTED to go out with him, which I no longer did. Had he had a great excuse or shown any expression of regret for being so late, I would have felt as if I mattered.

Once again those voices of my associates saying that I was too picky rang in my ears. So again I just swallowed my first reactions and said, "What kind of food are you interested in eating?" Knowing that I liked bland food, I added, "I liked simple cooking." Ben replied "Great let's go to Polly's Pies". Now I actually liked Polly's, but it was a far cry from any kind of restaurant that would have required a reservation. However, the coffee shop would be able to get us out quickly, if we wanted to try to make a show. We went out to his car and I was looking at a 1976 LeSabre. The fact that the car was twenty years old was not a concern. My concern came from how absolutely filthy the car looked, and how full of trash—fast food wrappers, tin cans, etc.—it was inside. That was quite another side of Ben that I had not expected. Ben hadn't made a clean place for me to sit, but he did open the car door. I quickly tried to brush the wrappers from the seat onto the floor. If he noticed, he made no comment of it. Nor did I. His choice of attire was drastically different from the outfit at the dance and lecture. He was wearing a pair of grass green dockers with a T-shirt with an emblem of a moose head that advertised some kind of beer on the back. He was wearing top sider shoes with no socks. My peach outfit was casual too. There was nothing wrong with the clothes that he was wearing, they simply did not leave the same impression as he had in the beginning. I quickly remembered that he had worn that great outfit at both places. Perhaps he only owned one fantastic outfit. Women usually had a larger selection of totally coordinated outfits hanging in their closets than men would have in theirs.

If I had been seeing someone for some time, it would be normal to get comfortable with their style of dressing and not put as much emphasis on it. But that was not how I perceived our situation. Perhaps Ben saw it differently. At Polly's the conversation was mainly about the big fight that was to take place in Las Vegas. Ben was all excited about the betting he had made on the outcome. Although I was not particularly a fight fan, I could have listened to details about it for about an hour. When it dominated a three-hour period, I had reached my saturation point and turned my ears off. It was clear that the idea of the movie had been erased from his memory. I wanted to erase this evening from mine. I was eager to return to my apartment. I wanted nothing more than to say goodnight in the car and to turn out the lights on the date.

Ben had other ideas. He never noticed that I was not really "there" as he rambled on and on and on. When we got back to my apartment, he wanted to come in. I tried to be polite and suggested that we make it a short night. Ben started to rebuff my suggestion, when he said "Oh OK, just let me use the little boys room before I get on the road." I saw no harm in that and we walked towards my apartment. I noticed my neighbor was home and made reference of it to Ben. When we got inside my apartment, I told him the bathroom was down the hall on the left. I went to the kitchen and got a glass of water. It seemed like Ben was in the bathroom a bit longer than I would have expected, but then sometimes Nature did require you to.

I went back into the living room and turned the TV on. Sitting in silence was not a comfortable idea to me. Twenty minutes had now passed, and I considered calling into the hall to make sure he was really

OK. It was much longer than the normal amount of time a man needed to "use the little boys room". Then Ben appeared, stark naked in the living room with his clothes rolled up under his right arm. I was shocked! I almost started to laugh because it seemed so absurd, when I noticed that his expression was **not** friendly at all. Perhaps I had seen too many TV movies about single women being attacked or raped while on a date, regardless that was not what I expected....

A little voice inside my head said to get out of there. But Ben would have been able to get to the front door long before I could have reached it. I immediately went to the kitchen to put space in between us. And that gave me a moment to think. The phone was in the bedroom and I did not want him in there! I needed a plan and I needed it immediately. I decided to stay calm and I reached for a glass and asked him if he would like a drink? Then I noticed I had a paring knife in the dish drainer, and grabbed it. I walked back into the living room with the knife pointed at his lower abdomen. In a slow, *but most forceful voice,* I told Ben to get out of my house or he would have a new life as a eunuch. My next door neighbor was a cop and he could have been there in seconds if I just screamed once. "Get the hell out of my house NOW!!!!" I screamed loudly. By the grace of God, Ben did just that.

The very next day, I called the organizer of the dance that I had attended. She was very concerned when weirdoes showed up at her events. They could have ruined her attendance and reputation very quickly. She said she would ban him from all future events. I only hoped that he had not raped anyone. Considering what could have happened to me while alone in my apartment, I was VERY lucky. It just reminded me how careful all single women have to be in our society today. You just could not always tell a wolf in sheep's clothing.

Story Seventeen: Single Mixers

Every weekend you can look in the accent section of the local newspaper to read what groups are planning a social event. Usually they have a small blurb about the activity and what the group does on a regular basis. Such a listing was in my local paper, "The Register's Accent section." Posted for the upcoming Saturday night were some interesting events. I was reading the announcement on Thursday. I was looking for things to do to that would have filled my weekend with other plans besides chores, videos, or reading. A small notice caught my eye about a singles group which promoted health awareness. The article was not very specific and did not even list the complete title of the group. Since it was concerned about health issues, perhaps they would hold a smoke-free form of entertainment. That was not easy to find these days. I called the number offered in the paper. It was a pre-recorded message, and the information was sketchy at best. The mixer was to be held at the prestigious Crown's Sterling hotel. The directions were easy to follow. What the heck, I did not have much else planned so I decided to try it out. Besides I had never been inside that five star hotel, and felt that that alone would be worth the trip.

On Saturday night, I closed the salon around four p.m. That gave me time to have my hair and makeup refreshed and change my clothes. Since I had never attended the group's events before, I decided to dress extra conservatively. I selected a light tan dress made of rayon. It was mid-calf in length and long-sleeved and it fit so well that I actually looked thinner when I wore it. The dress also had tiny pearls sewn on the collar and cuffs. Women often have a "favorite outfit" in their closets, that was mine.

The mixer was called for 5:30 p.m. and so I arrived at 6 p.m. I wanted to get there early enough to find a good "spot" that would allow me to watch the goings on. With a new group, I had found it best not to be one of the first to arrive. I decided a half-hour was a good choice.

Feeling that my presentation was OK, I walked into the hotel lobby where the group was to meet. From the moment I walked through the electronic doors, a lot of commotion could be heard. It sounded like it was a happening place, and I felt exhilarated. There was a large crowd already gathered around the piano lounge.

As I got closer to the crowd I noticed a unique pattern was established. The group was largely male. These men were gorgeous to look at, they could all have been models for men's fashions. For a second, I actually thought that might have been a convention of men that all worked in the fashion industry. After all, hotels were known to hold meetings and conferences for many different kinds of businesses. Then there were some women all cloistered together off to one side. They were dramatic looking, with black leather clothing, very short crew-cuts and hair colors of vivid shades of red, blue, and black. I immediately felt that I looked out of place with these people. The women were deep into conversation with each other, and hadn't noticed me at all. Given how ridiculously out of place I felt, that was fine. I let my eyes roam the room. I wasn't able see anyone else in the lounge who looked like the typical single I was used to seeing at other mixers. Most of the men had their arms around each other in a very casual but familiar way. I began to wonder if this was a gay and lesbian group.

I went up to the bartender and asked if this was where the Singles Mixer was to meet? He nodded and said they are all here for the same group. My sense of disappointment must have been easy to recognize. The man simply said: "Perhaps this isn't the kind of mixer you expected." By the tone of his voice I could tell it wasn't a question but rather a polite way of being told that I was not going to fit in.

On my way out of the hotel lobby, I stopped by the bell captain's stand and asked if there was another singles mixer scheduled anywhere else in the hotel. It was confirmed that there were none. I glanced down at the list of hotel meeting groups and saw the name of the group that was meeting in the piano lounge. It read "The Boy's Club—Single's Mixer and Swap Hop." Obviously the newspaper had left out that important information when it listed the event. The group may have been interested in health issues that I would have agreed were important. But that evening all I wanted to do was be amongst the same kind of people that I would have wanted to date. As I drove home, I stopped by my local video rental and picked out three oldies but goodies. It was going to be a long weekend after all.

Chapter Fourteen

Dining and Dieting

Story Eighteen: The Tootsie Roll Diet

I have first-hand knowledge of the power of dieting. I have tried so many of them that I could write a book about the diets and their false promises. The key word most of us have forgotten in the word D-I-E-T is *DIE*. That is what we are forced to deal with when we just blindly jump into a current diet craze. People learn of them from the media and from their friends. No one means to harm us. We don't want to harm our selves. But we do, and we spend billions of dollars each year in the search for the *perfect body*.

The simple truth that took me thirty years to truly understand was, **I would *NEVER* have the perfect body if I compared it to anyone else's!!!** I simply had to get my brain to accept that I had the best body *for me*. The last sentence was a lot easier to type than it was to believe!!! Finally I had. I always needed to be careful as I watched what I ate. For I would always have the tendency to want to eat too many sugary sweets and bread type foods. Even in moderation, I would never have made the cover of any magazine, I would, however, have a closet full of beautiful clothes that I enjoyed to wear.

Everyone knows that exercise is essential to stay healthy. But what happens if the usual aerobic programs cause you to burst into tears? The key is to find just one thing that you really like to do and do it often. For me it's dancing. Therefore, I made an effort and did some form of dance four times a week. There were added benefits to that kind of workout, ie: the socializing could be terrific too. Health clubs, and exercise gyms design their entire workouts to be more social and lure young applicants. Co-ed step and aerobic classes make the atmosphere feel more like a party then a work out for the participants. I have worked in several different fitness centers. I watched the socializing as it went on and it usually amused me.

Many of the women who came in looked as though they just came from the salon with their hair and makeup fully done. Their workout clothes looked like they just came from the dry cleaners. And they wore much too much perfume. I did not care what brand you used or how much you paid for it, when you mix body perspiration with heavy perfume odors, it simply created a stronger stink! That was particularly true for men.

Most fitness centers are wall-to-wall mirrors. I often stood back and observed these people watching themselves in these mirrors, it was always interesting. I had designed a system where I categorized the attendees into two areas, the real exercisers, and the workout players. I could spot them instantly when they walked into the door. Although all of the fitness centers that I had worked in had never set these two groups apart, I felt that it would have done them both a better service. The people that were really interested in working their muscles were more likely to have enjoyed sharing the same gym space with those that had the same goals.

Most health clubs have a limited number of machines. When a customer came in to just "hang out," they would waste time on the equipment. The serious exerciser would want to get on and off more efficiently. With both customers working out at the same time, the availability of equipment was compromised. The serious jock was usually not interested in idle chatter or gossip. The conversations, between those opposing customers, were difficult. I had watched them many times and it was uncomfortable. I had suggested that schedules could be offered for "serious workout times" and "social gathering sessions". The concept had merit, however, implementing it would have been hard to do. The management had trouble determining what would have been a fair and equitable split.

Another part of the gym routine that was very un-balanced, was the music that was played. Everyone agreed the music should have a lively, pulsating beat. But the lyrics were most often degrading to women. I would have loved to hear the women's song about a man's body! Let the men in the club work out while a *female* singer was crooning out words like "gimme that ass of yours oh baby", "Pump it up tonight", "I have something hard for you". Where did the fitness centers get those awful songs???

Besides the social aspect of the gym, there were fitness reasons that brought women to join. Women should remember whatever muscle mass they developed when they were thirty, would be harder to maintain when they were forty. During the aging process, muscles lost tone and then atrophied. When that occurred, the body looked less desirable than when it had too much fat on it. Whatever anyone thought about the appearance of fat, flabby muscles were less esthetically appealing. A lot of women were very **weight** conscious. They painfully weighed in every day. The process was self-destructing. Muscle mass weighed a lot more than fat. The more you worked out, the heavier your total body weight would have been. My suggestion was to throw away the scale and let the mirror be the guide. IF you liked what you saw, then you should have enjoyed it!

Several years ago, I read a report done on the psychological evaluation of men's and women's reactions to their appearance. One hundred men and women were asked "Did they think they were good-looking?" All one hundred men said yes. Ninety-nine women offered their personal critique of their bodies, beginning with what ever element or feature that they felt they most lacked. One woman started to say yes and then quickly changed into the pattern of the others.

All of these two hundred volunteers were interviewed separately so that their responses were not influenced by the others' answers. The men decided that they had to answer affirmatively, the alternative was not an acceptable consideration. Whereas the women could not bring them-selves to think that they were good-looking. Boy our society sure has gotten things skewed off balance.

Fads and dieting seemed to go hand in hand. The Grapefruit Diet, The Watermelon Diet, The Three Day Fasting Diet, The Chicken Noodle Diet, whatever you wanted to call it, someone has probably conjured it up. For every fad there were thousands of gullible people who tried it. The real harm in fad dieting was the roller coaster ups and downs of the scale. We tend to lose the ten to twenty pounds only later to have put **back on** twenty to thirty pounds! Similar to the performance of the toy yo-yo, our bodies stretched and shrunk continually. Added to the equa-tion, the normal aging process and it's effect on the body, and we had a real dilemma.

Society has been full of obese men and women. Statistics reflected the trend that all children in the US were at a greater risk of obesity than at any other time in history. With all the emphasis that was placed on looking "**perfect**", it seemed particularly ironic that the trend was going in the opposite direction for the next generation. Isn't it time we enjoyed a "Tootsie roll" as a tiny piece of candy and not a monumental lifestyle crisis.

Story Nineteen: Romantic Dining With An Extra Ten Pounds

For all of you that could relate to the effort of reducing a few pounds, you would be able to appreciate what a single woman goes through trying to date and keep to a diet. Personally I was thrilled with the movie *"When Harry Met Sally"*. Meg Ryan played a character that specialized every entree she ordered in any restaurant. Ex.: She would order an item without the sauce, or some other dish without salt, etc. I found myself relating to the need to customizing dinners. As I watched her on the big screen I became so uplifted but also confused. Meg made it seem so easy, but when I tried it I only got dirty looks from the waiter/ waitress. I finally decided that it was just easier to cook at home, and then to go out on a date.

I wouldn't have felt comfortable suggesting that I cooked dinner on a first date. It would be better to have gotten to know someone first, before they were invited into my home. After all, there were some risks any woman might take in the beginning of any dating relationship. On the side of caution, a woman should have her first date be in a public place. I had met a man named Mac. He said he was in his late forties, however his leathery skin and very thin hair made him appear to be in his late fifties. Since women have been known to exaggerate their ages, why shouldn't a man be able to do the same? Mac was 5'5' and very slight build. Honestly I thought I could have possibly out weighed him by ten pounds. Even though his face looked weather-beaten, he had a warm, friendly appearance. The one major drawback, were the lobster-style claws he had for hands. I couldn't imagine how computer sales-man got hands in that condition. The only profession that came to my mind would have been a long-shoreman. Mac had the most wonderful stories to tell. He kept me in stitches with all the antics he could relate....Conversations with him were always delightful and most often very colorful. It was after our third date, that I decided to offer Mac a home-cooked meal. He loved to go out to eat and especially to exotic restaurants. I ate very plain, mildly seasoned food. I actually preferred foods that were bland rather than spicy. It was a Friday night. Because I worked early on Saturdays, it would have forced us to have a short evening. It has been my experience that dates were better if they were shorter. Wanting to spend more time together was more enjoyable than counting the minutes until it was over. Even though I had had several other dates with Mac, I still wanted to keep an at-home dinner date short. I also wanted to go out afterwards, rather than just to hang out in my living room.

From my personal experience, one major drawback of offering to cook for a man, was the chance that he would not have wanted to just "stay in" after the dinner was completed. Or worse would have been if the man tried to make unwanted sexual passes.... On all the other dates, no unwanted advances had been made. It was why I had suggested dinner at my place. I thought I was dealing with a nice well-mannered man. Previously, he offered assistance getting in and out of his car. Would offer to let me be seated before he did, and would rise when I got up from the table. His manners were perfect. Although there was an inner sense in my head that made me feel that he might have been putting most of it on for show. I dismissed my doubts, and spent no time worrying about it. I was certain he would be a gentleman.

Deciding to cook dinner for him solved two problems. I wanted to eat more blandly and Mac ate out all the time. A home cooked meal would be a refreshing change, and a saving to his wallet too. Mac had told me that he would eat all three meals a day in restaurants, five out of seven days. I thought a home cooked meal was just what he might have liked, to break the tradition.

During conversations on the other dates, glimpses of his home life were revealed. Mac had come from the lower east side of Brooklyn. He had had some tough and rough experiences in his growing up years. Perhaps his hands got so abused back then, that they were still so beaten up. Mac didn't drink to an access, but by the end of the other dates, his speech was slightly affected by the alcohol. He had made one reference to the fact that he felt a home was a place for comfort and not to have been a show place. Although he never mentioned it, I assumed that at home, Mac would be a beer and nuts kind of a man rather than wine and cheese. I created a dinner to fill the comfort zone he was used too, but would not have made him so comfortable that he would have "rolled off the couch".

As I had already stated, I was forever fighting the bulge. I considered serving turkey, since it was a low fat food, which would fit the reduced fat requirement. However, its tricophene made me sluggish. Tricophene was the natural hormone in turkeys that made them so docile. I had to cross that off the list. I decided on fresh fish.

Because of the aroma that fish created, I liked to use an outdoor barbecue. Living in Southern California allowed me to use a barbecue year round. Wrapping the fish in foil made clean-up a breeze. I took fresh lemon slices and laid them all over the top of the fish. I used Old Bay and Spike for seasonings. With all fish dishes, rice compliments them well. I loved potatoes, but they were too tempting to top with the "fat goodies….butter, sour cream, or cheese." I could blend wild and white rice with fat-free broth instead of water, and got a good flavorful rice dish without a lot of calories. To round it all out, I added steamed carrots and broccoli seasoned with Spike plus a dash of lemon and orange juices. The blend of seasoned rice and veggies with the fish was a hearty meal without feeling like I had gone off my diet. Added touches that did not add too many calories were as follows:

As an appetizer:

I mixed one half a head of Boston / butter lettuce, one can of Mandarin Orange slices, one tablespoon slivered almonds and one tablespoon of raisins. I tossed and sprinkled one heaping teaspoon of fat free dill salad dressing over the dish.

For the dessert:

There was always something about a smooth, creamy texture that left a sensuous feel. I loved creamy desserts but couldn't have had the fat or calories. For years I felt deprived. Then Jell-O® came out with fat-free, sugar free puddings. Once you mixed it with skim milk, the end result was heavenly. I mixed into it, swirls of fat-free chocolate toppings and then a single strawberry rested on the very top of the parfait glass. That made a beautiful looking dessert that was low-cal too.

I also liked to add music to the event. I pre-selected mood music for the entire meal from a list of CD's. I programmed the player before Mac arrived. I started with New Age work from Yanni, then I added John Tesh. After the mellow sounds of these two, I kicked up the tempo to Melloncamp, Earth Wind and Fire, and Bryan Adams. When dessert was to be served, I wanted a more sensuous mood to go with the luscious feel of the parfait. I chose Celine Dion and Barbra Streisand.

Lighting was the final touch. Candles were on the dining room table but not lit. In the lamps in the living room I placed twenty-five watt bulbs. I had two lamps and I selected a soft pink bulb for one and a light blue for the other. As women aged, lighting was an important tool that created the right look. If asked, any leading lady in a movie would have agreed......

Scents were also important. If I were not so concerned with calories, I would have baked a cake. The smell of fresh baked goods was really the BEST scent to impress any man. I chose a drop of my own perfume to be placed on the wire rim on the lamp shade. When the light bulb warmed the metal, the scent filled the air. Shalimar was the perfume I had loved for decades. The vanilla extract in its formula brought wonderful responses from men. Time would tell if Mac liked it too.

I carefully planned my outfit. Since I was the hostess, I wanted to make sure that I didn't look like I was ready for bed. Nor did I want to look like I was just wearing any old thing. After rummaging through my entire closet, I selected a simple black silk dress. I decided not to wear any jewelry, to make sure that I did not look too dressed up.

From my experience, men loved long flowing hair on women, and Mac was no exception. Therefore, I used hot rollers and gave volume and style to my long hair and wore it down. After retouching my makeup, I was ready for Mac's arrival. So I thought....

Everyone has pet peeves, mine was with punctuality. With cooking fish, timing was extremely important. I even confirmed the time earlier in the day. Mac said he would be at my apartment at seven sharp. It was already seven forty-five and I had not heard from him. Part of me was worried that he might have had car trouble or even worse, an accident. Not hearing from him, my mind went back and forth from anger to worry and back again. I really wished he had called. Knowing was better than speculation.

As the clock chimed half past eight, Mac knocked on my door. I tried to stay calm as he sauntered into my living room. "Hi babe, what's for dinner? I'm starved," he said nonchalantly. He was wearing a blue Izod pullover shirt, and gray cotton pants. Casual and comfortable would best describe his appearance, but it gave no indication where he might have been taking me after dinner. If I had wanted to analyze it, I would have realized that it meant he wanted to go nowhere that evening. I was too miffed to think about much of anything, except his rudeness.

I had learned to count to ten before I verbally lashed out. In my head I recited 1, 2, 3,... Because I was not sure how my anger might have surfaced, I kept very quiet. Anger has been known to dilate many peoples' pupils. In the past I knew mine had been affected that way when I was angry. I was certain they would be like saucers. I kept my head tilted as if to be looking at the floor, just so that Mac would not be able to see how annoyed I was over his lateness.

The date was just starting and something inside of me felt obligated to try to make it enjoyable. I told him to sit down and asked what he would like to drink, moving toward the kitchen to check on dinner. I got the beverages. Mid-way to the kitchen, he called after me, "Get me a brooskie and pass on the glass." Somehow my ears registered the latter part of that request as "AND PISS ON THE GLASS". I wanted to say "you deserve nothing better you asshole," but instead I just said, "Excuse me, what was that last part?" Mac replied "Don't bother with a glass." He preferred the beer straight up. I came back into the living room with the beer and a coaster. Maybe he would use it if I placed the beer bottle on it first. "You said you were hungry, so we can begin with the appetizers any time you're ready," I said half-heartedly. Mac responded that he had hoped that it wasn't going to be some fancy dinner. He got his fill of those at restaurants. He was looking forward to some down home meat and potatoes and of course with beer. Mac complimented me on my selection of beer, he thought it was a good one. "Where did you find it?" he inquired. I told him at Trader Joe's the beer was being promoted there. Than I added: "Glad you liked it." I did not think the dinner was at all fancy. The menu consisted of fish, rice and fresh veggies. I chose a thresher shark because it tasted more like chicken than fish. I thought he might have liked it. Mac retorted: "Naw, couldn't say that I have eaten much fish. Ever since I saw the movie Jaws, I haven't thought much of sharks."

Well now I felt like I was in a tight spot. This was what I had for dinner and I was not looking to throw it out. So I timidly said, "How about if you tried a small amount of my dinner, you might find out that you liked it." I thought that was a good idea, and the least he could do since I had tried to make a nice dinner just for him. Mac must **not** have agreed because he said "Why don't we chuck the fish and order a large pizza?" Unfortunately, even if I felt compelled to oblige his request, I was very allergic to the ingredients in pizza, mainly the cheese, tomatoes and onions. Well that was the *last* straw. I was not going to throw out all of my food. So I just turned to face him directly and said, "Look Mac, my home is NOT a restaurant." I had worked hard to plan and cook that dinner. And I was going to eat it with or without his help. He could have decided to be a decent dinner guest and politely tried my cooking or he could have gotten the hell out of my house! If pizza was what he wanted there was a Pizza Hut right down the street.

I was sure my pupils were dilated, my nostrils flared and my temper was past being able to be contained. I decided it was not worth trying to save the date. After all, he was so late without a word about it. And his cockiness about the food plus he had an air about him that made me feel like I was a waitress in my own home, rather than his dinner companion. He glared at me and with more balls than a bull would have had told me "Well babe, it was my loss because dessert was going to be in the bedroom and he could have made me creme like I had never done before." I was so shocked, I was certain my face showed it. He had *never shown this side* of him before on the other three dates.

That did it! If I had the tiniest bit of guilt that I was ending the date too soon, I was certain that I had made the right decision then. That would have been just one more man that felt that dinner at home meant dessert was served in the bedroom....

CHAPTER FIFTEEN

Unique Experiences for
A Single Woman

Story Twenty: Libations, Inhibitions, and Vacations

The sense of freedom was one of the best parts about traveling to a new place. The increased willingness to break out of normal behavior, was a major part of that freedom. People did things they might never had considered appropriate at home. Many people would have said that not having to worry about what other people thought of them, aided the exploration along. The carefree action seemed acceptable, because no one was forced to explain their behavior to strangers.

Cruise ships and single travel groups created special drinks that were served to their guests just to let their inhibitions loose. Hypnotists are often hired to entertain the "troupes" just so that their inner *wild-side* could be enjoyed by the group. For many people just getting away from normal routines would have brought it out too.

I had a close friend from college, named Joan. I was an accounting major back then and Joan majored in European History. Ultimately she wanted to become a teacher or a librarian. Joan did become a librarian. I did not make it in the world of "debits, credits and liabilities". She was always quite and shy. I was not a loud person, but by comparison, I was definitely more outgoing. We made good traveling companions. Our strengths complimented each other. Although we got along very well, we certainly looked like opposites. Joan was 5'9" in bare feet with lanky legs, blonde hair and blue eyes and a porcelain complexion. Whereas I was the short 5'2", stocky one with olive skin and brown-black eyes and dark brown hair. Nobody would have ever mistook us as sisters.

Joan and I decided to take a trip to Europe. We planned for a whole year. She took some brief classes in Italian and German at a local Junior college. I tried to bone up on my French by purchasing the learn-at-home tape programs. I was not sure how well they would have worked, but it made driving in the car more enjoyable. After careful planning and re-scheduling a few dozen times, we selected London/England, Paris/France, and Rome/Italy as our travel itinerary.

We understood we were following the most traveled tourist program and it did not sound particularly challenging. However, since we were new at international travel, we thought it best to stick to areas that were known for their tourist appeal. England would be our first stop. Joan had her heart set on Bed and Breakfasts instead of hotels. She felt that they would give us a sense of "local color" that a hotel chain would not have offered. It didn't matter one way or the other to me. An English pub had such an arrangement. The place was out in the country. We took a hanson ride to the pub once we reached the city. Unlike taxi service in the states, the fare was arranged at the time of arrival and was a flat fee. That made it very enjoyable to sit back and let the horse and carriage take us to where we had to go. Many of the streets were cobblestones and the horse's hooves bumped us along.

Joan was not prone to motion sickness, I had to fight falling to sleep for the jostling. The countryside was magnificent. The rich foliage and rolling hills were more beautiful than words could describe. Once we were at the pub, the caretaker showed us to our rooms. The furniture was antique looking. Although my tastes ran more to the modern style, seeing the antiques in a setting that fit them, made the room look luxurious. I noticed that there was no toilet in the room. We were told it was down the hall and that everyone on that floor shared it. My sense of privacy and sanitation bristled a bit but other than that the accommodations were lovely.

Every evening we were invited to dine on fish and chips and drink with the locals. Since we were so far from the center of town, that made a lot of sense. Even though the language was supposed to be the same, we felt like we were in a foreign land as we listened to their accents and expressions. We noticed how they liked to party.

The pub was lively as early as four p.m. and it did not close until six a.m. We took naps from the jet lag and the long journey from New York. When we awoke, we quickly freshened up using the wash bowl in our room. We changed our traveling clothes and slipped into gauzy multi-printed skirts and white, cotton peasant blouses. We sort of had a Sophia Loren look going on. Our reflections in the graying, antiqued mirror pleased us. As we set off to find the tavern, we could hear the raucous from our doorway. All the while the laughter and carrying on was contagious.

On the very first night, Joan got on top of the bar and sang at the top of her lungs. I was taken by surprise by her behavior. It was such a diversion from the way she would have normally acted. As I said before, I was considered the more gregarious one. I couldn't have remembered a single time that she had initiated any conversation with the strangers we would encounter, now this! Joan's surprised outburst was a mixture based on how the pub's ale effected her and really *bad* singing.

As much as I adored her, singing was **not** her special gift. The locals seemed not to mind. Several pitched right in and their voices were no more melodic as a group than Joan's had been as a solo. Then the entertainment went from songs to a challenged game of some sort.

When it became your turn, if you could not come up with the words to the song, you were forced to chug-a-lug a bottle of beer, or you did a shooter of bourbon. Either one would have made you pretty sauced. I had not seen Joan drink more than two mixed drinks in an entire evening. Currently she had lost three consecutive rounds, and had downed three shooters by the time I made my way to the bar. I called out to Joan. I thought it was time to go back to our rooms. We had an early departure for France the next day. There was no doubt in my mind that the train ride would be better without a severe hangover. Joan slurred her response, so I knew I was in for a rough night and possibly a hard morning. In a sing song style, she attempted to call after me: "You're a party pooper. Every party needs a pooper, that's why we invited YOU, Party-Pooper." Then the whole pub chimed in "Party-pooper, Party-pooper, which really sounded like they were singing Parr-dee Pop-per, Parr-dee Pop-per.

I knew when to quit. I just turned on my heels and went up to our assigned room. I was awakened several hours later, to the sound of Joan's retching over the porcelain pitcher. As I mentioned before, the bed and breakfast pub accommodated each guest with their own room not their own bath. That was down the hall. Obviously, Joan hadn't made it that far. At first I was still annoyed at her stupid antics, from earlier in the evening. I figured she got her *just rewards*. But soon afterwards, it was clear that she was really miserable. I got up and tended to her needs. Joan promised that she would not repeat her performance for the rest of her life. I told her if she tried to keep her promise until the end of the trip that would be long enough for me. Once we were back to the States, I would no longer have felt responsible for her. Then whatever she wanted to do would be A-OK with me.

Story Twenty-one: Oh La-La, Words of Love Are So Much More Exciting In A Foreign Language

When Joan and I arrived in Paris, we were tired, hungry and covered in soot from the long train ride. We had gotten a euro-rail pass so that we could ride the trains from one country to the other. Our blue jeans and pink sweat-shirts looked black and mauve after the soot settled in the fibers. We went right to our second B&B. It's location was more ideal than the last, and we would be able to take the Paris subway from it's front door to the center of the city. All we wanted was a clean room with two great, comfortable beds so that we might have slept for ten hours. In reality, the room was simple and just OK. It had no antiques, just two twin beds and a chair and table. The bath was right next door and we only had to share it with one other tourist. Tthe mattresses were so soft, they felt like pillows instead of a mattress, and we had six hours left to shower, eat (if we wanted) and sleep. We both opted to skip the showers until the next morning. We decided to go for a small snack at the bistro across the way. And then last but not least, we'd have slept on the floor if the "pillow-like" mattresses turned out to be useless. We knew we'd feel better with our stomachs full, and headed for the bistro. We quickly changed our clothes. Joan put on a black turtle necked jersey and white linen trousers. I wore a white sweater and black gabardine black slacks. We enjoyed looking like opposite bookends. After all we were in the world's fashion capital, the perfect place to have made a fashion statement.

Jean-Val Claude was our waiter. He could have just stepped out of the cover a French GQ magazine. He was so tall that he made Joan look short! I would have looked ridiculous if I stood next to him. His hair was straight, thick and jet black, and so were his large saucer shaped eyes. He had the most perfect face, either of us had ever seen. I ordered cafe laits for both of us and two croissants filled with fete cheese. Normally, I did not like goat's cheese, but right then I was too hungry or tired to care. Jean-Val Claude knew immediately that we were Americans and tried to speak English with us. He invited us to meet his cousin for dinner and dancing. How or what possessed us to agree, I could not have explained. It defied all logic.

There we were, our first night in Paris, and we were seated in a crowded cafe style club, as loud sultry French music played in the background. Even with my attempts of learning French, the words to the music made no sense. The singer made the works sound very suggestive and romantic. Jean -Val Claude and his cousin Henri had kissed our fingertips, nibbled on our necks and earlobes and whispered what was probably the equivalent of "French nothings" into our ears. Somehow it did not seem inconsequential that evening. Henri was not as attractive as his cousin, but still looked nice. Henri stood around 5'10". He had the same beautiful hair and dark eyes. It must have been a family trait both men had inherited. Because of the differences in height, Jean-Val was paired off with Joan and Henri was my chosen companion.

We both thought it was fantastic. Joan and I no longer felt tired or glum. We danced and kissed into the wee hours of the morning. When we finally got back to our marshmallow mattresses, neither of us gave a hoot. We were already floating on clouds anyway. Before we left the cafe, Joan and I promised to write to the young men. We left the next morning for a full day of sight seeing. The owner of the B&B was an elder man with thinning white hair and laughing, crinkly eyes. Monsieur Robert (pronounced like Row-bear) had packed us a boxed lunch of smoked cheeses, baguettes, fresh picked oranges and grapes, slices of ham, chicken and lamb and quarter pieces of tomatoes, cucumber, and a bottle of white wine to take with us. It was a good thing we had traveled light, the weight of our lunch was considerable. It was so kind of Monsieur Robert, we graciously accepted. We started out in the direction of the city's metro. Just as we were half way down the road, a car horn honked at us. Joan and I were immediately surprised to see Jean and Henri in a blue, older model Mercedes Benz sedan. They had taken their other cousin's car so they could be our tour guides for the afternoon.

We thought we would be seeing the Louvre museum, the Effel tower, and several other famous tourist spots on our list. The young men had other plans. We spent the most wonderful day with them, as we explored the nooks and crannies of the "real" city. Jean and Henri took us to a magnificent restaurant for a traditional French dinner, which was eaten in the late afternoon. We tried to tell them that we had enough food in our "boxed lunches" for all of us. They wouldn't hear of it, and insisted that we were their guest for the day. Neither of us wanted to upset them, so we placed the boxes in the trunk of the sedan. The aromas that greeted us at the front door told us we were in for some special treat. The food was rich and delicious. There were creamy sauces on just about everything. From the asparagus tips to the chateau breion, the sauces were divine. Fresh fruits with slices of cheese were served between each course. After six courses, I decided it was best to stop counting. My diet was blown for the whole year on just that one dinner. But what a way to go! In Paris it was customary for a light supper to be served at the end of the day. Unlike in the states, we would have eaten a light lunch and a bigger dinner. When in Paris, we did as they did. Afterwards, Jean and Henri brought us back to their place. It was not far from our B &B. To compare their living quarters to apartments back home, it would have been considered a studio size with one extra loft attached. They did have a private bathroom with an old fashioned porcelain tub on four legs (no shower). Although there wasn't any visible signs of an actual bedroom, they had two futons that opened to accommodate them. We were romanced in the truest sense of the word back at Jean's and Henri's flat.

By Joan's and my account, Paris was the City Of Love!!!!

Story Twenty-two: Single-hood and the Holidays

Everywhere you turn there were advertisements about families and the holidays. Gatherings for grandparents, aunts, uncles and cousins, and of course moms, dads and the kids. With the national divorce rate higher than fifty percent, where were ads about extended families and children with only one parent? And how about the baby boomer generation that did not get married and lived alone? Where were the advertisements for them? Was living alone supposed to be considered some form of torture?

From a personal perspective, I did not think of it as torture or any form of punishment. I loved the freedom it allowed. Here was just a partial list of all the things you could do if you lived alone:

1. Living alone gave you an ability to explore self-indulgent behavior with no risk of guilt.

2. There was always no waiting for the bathroom. If at the last minute you remembered a party you had been invited to, you could have gotten ready quickly. You also had the freedom of having plenty of hot water for a gorgeously luxurious hot soak or long shower.

3. You could have played whatever music you felt like enjoying. You did not have to feel compelled to listen to just holiday caroling. In addition, you could play your music at any hour of the day. The volume control was all up to you.

4. If you were expecting guests over, you could clean your home/condo or apartment in the nude.

5. You could have eaten a frozen dinner entree right out of the package while you watched TV and no one would ever have known it.

6. You could have eaten your dessert before eating your vegetables without being told it would have made you fat, or ruined your appetite.

7. The relatives would not have expected you to "house" the holiday gathering because your place would have usually been smaller than the others. After all, living alone hadn't required you to have four bedrooms and three bathrooms with a dining table to seat twelve adults.

8. You would be asked to bring a dish of something for the family meal, but most often you wouldn't be asked to make the main course. That allowed your grocery bill to remain within the normal range of your household expenses instead of your already tight budget being ruined.

9. As a single person, you could have gotten out of accepting an invitation to a family party , if you said that you had a "date". Most of your married relatives eagerly wanted you to find that "special person" that would put an end to your Single-hood.

10. Being single also gave you a good excuse for not baby-sitting every weekend for your nieces/ nephews. Your sibling(s) may have wanted to go out with their spouse(s) but not if your chance to be with "Mr./Miss Right" would be destroyed.

11. You could have talked on the phone all night long without having to whisper so as not to have awakened anybody else.

12. You would always have found that piece of pie you left in the refrigerator. And no one else would have had to know if you woke up at 3:00 am. and wanted to finish it.

13. You could have surfed the channels on the TV remote and no one would have told you to stop.

14. Your video tape player could have recorded all of your favorite shows and then you could have watched them at your leisure.

With all the above-mentioned good things about being alone, there were some problems with it on the holidays. I lived in Southern California and all my relatives lived on the East coast, Virginia and Florida respectively. Going back to Virginia during the winter was not my idea of a wise decision. I had gotten use to warm weather all year round. Therefore cold, blustery or snowy weather was not inviting. Florida would be a good choice but since winter was the SnowBirds season, the flight prices were very high. Thus I stayed put for the holidays. If you turned on the TV, listened to the radio, or read a newspaper, you could not have missed all the presentations about the holidays were for being with your family. That started to wear on my nerves after a while.

Like a lot of the other singles, I was invited to go to friends' families for the holidays. Over the years, I had accepted many such invitations. The trouble with sharing with nice strangers was that no matter how nice they were, they were not really related to you. They could not replace your own family. They gathered around telling about all the funny events that had happened to them through the years, and you politely listened. For me, it just conjured up my own memories and made me "homesick".

Sometimes after a few social cocktails, the alcohol could unleash the "tiger" in one or more of your friend's relatives. The conversation could change to a more cantankerous style. Believe me, as an outsider, that was not any easier to witness. Being single and unattached at the holi-days made me desire to hook up with a partner. Then I would have had the celebration with a new "*significant other.*" For all of you that were single at the holidays, I would have wished for you, just such an event.

Story Twenty-three: Baseball The American Favorite Pastime

I had to admit that I was not much of a sports fan. I barely knew enough to tell the difference from a right fielder and a lineman. Besides one being on a baseball team and the other on a football field, I could not have won any points on a trivial pursuit game. For I had not attempted to make myself more familiar with America's favorite pastime sports. Yet every time I tried to watch them on TV, I got so mixed up or bored that I fell asleep. Perhaps growing up without any brothers may have contributed to some of my lack of knowledge, matched with a lack of enthusiasm.

Things were going to change. I decided to try to get into the groove and learn about baseball. A single Season ticket was given as a raffled door prize at one charity event I decided to attend. As many singles would attest too, last minute plans were part of the territory. Such was the case with my attending the charity dinner.

Arriving at the tale end of the cocktail hour, I was asked to participate in the drawing. My ticket may have been closer to the top of the barrel in order for me to be the winner. I certainly was not one who thought it was "good luck" that brought me to become the owner of the ticket. I took a moment to decide if I should have turned it over to someone else. Then I realized that it would have provided the ideal opportunity to learn about the game.

Living in Orange County I had to drive into Los Angeles country to the Dodgers Stadium, which was not an easy feat. Determined to meet my own goal, I wound up trekking through horrendous traffic to six games.

For the first game, I sat and watched everything. The people around my seat all seemed very preoccupied with the game. I was hoping to have found someone at the stadium that would have explained what I was watching. Sometimes I understood what the fuss was all about and a lot of the time I felt like a foreigner in a foreign land. Everyone spoke what seemed to be a strange language. I went home after the first game, with little understanding about baseball.

In the middle of the second game, I met Harry at the concession stand. He had purchased beer and a hot dog and I got a soda and a pretzel. He looked about seventy. His posture was poor, but he probably once stood at around six feet tall. Although all gray, his hair was still very wavy. His skin was leathery from being over-exposed to the sun. He really did look old. Harry had kind eyes, and when he asked me where I was seated, it turned out his place was two up from mine. I explained how little I knew about baseball but had won my seasons ticket. Immediately he offered to explain the game and gave me a few pointers. I gladly accepted. We walked back to our seats and my lessons began.

Harry may have been old and looked it most of the time, but when he got all excited in a game, then his face filled with boyish charm. It was really quite remarkable to watch the transformation. One minute he could look like a shriveled version of Walter Mathau, and then the game would get started and the bases were loaded, and he became a thirty year old version of Walter. Harry was a real sports enthusiast. He told me that he had seasons passes for the last forty-five years, and had never missed a home game. I believed him. Harry loved the game and was a terrific coach about the sport of baseball.

I would spring for his beers and hot-dogs, while he told me what was going on. Most of the time Harry had his own slant on what were happening, and his stories made the game seem more important. Each game would last several hours, and it amazed me how many beers he had put away. The alcohol never seemed to affect him. Still concerned, I asked him if he drove home from the stadium. He said he took the bus, so I figured it was OK to have kept the tab going. After all, I got the lessons I wanted and he got his refreshments free. He made it fun and I actually had begun to enjoy watching baseball.

By the fifth game, I looked forward to going to the stadium and meeting Harry. I hadn't noticed at the time, but he wore a different kind of outfit. For all the other games, he had worn sans a pan polyester pants, a T-shirts and baseball cap. That day he wore a faded leisure suit. I paid no attention to his appearance. Looking back at it, I should have. The game went into overtime and we both were excited about how it was fairing. I still did not care who won, but Harry sure did. The game ended with the Red Sox beating the Dodgers by one run. I thought it went well. Harry was upset and his mood changed. If I had known any better, I would have said he was a sorry-sport or a bad loser. Neither idea appealed to me, I guess I just did not have that competitive sporting side in me. Anyway, it began to rain. And I meant it was a really downpour. I did not want to see Harry standing out in the pouring rain as he waited for a late bus. I offered to drive him home. Luckily I had found a parking space closer to the entrance than usual. Since it hadn't looked like rain when the game started, I hadn't brought my umbrella. We ran to my red Toyota Corolla with newspapers over our heads in a futile attempt to stay dry. We were marginally soaked by the time we reached my car. Once the engine warmed up, I turned the heater on to help dry us out. I hadn't wanted either of us to catch a cold or flu. Although, I never learned Harry's true age, he was definitely a senior citizen, and they tended to be more susceptible to colds. In moments we were off to his house.

By that time, I had felt comfortable with Harry and did not mind going out of my way to have taken a friend home. He had gladly accepted my invitation to be his chauffeur. Then I realized that I did not have a clue to where he might have actually lived. I guess I jumped to the conclusion that if anyone took the local bus to get around that they must have lived somewhere in the neighborhood. Again my logic was all-wrong. It turned out that Harry lived in a section of Long Beach that was not an area for a young single girl to be caught out in, late at night. I could not have changed my mind and not taken him home. I was simply stuck carrying out my offer. Harry was still in his bad mood. I had bad feelings about the neighborhood, as we drove off to parts unknown.

Traffic in LA was bad anyway, but the rain made it worse. We started out at ten-thirty at night, and by midnight, we were still not at his house. I was not sure of my way around Long Beach. What I quickly learned was since Harry took the bus, he did not need to know all the streets. All passengers relied on the bus driver knowing how he got from one place to another. By twelve fifteen, I wanted to stop for directions, but Harry refused.

There must be something universal about men not wanting to admit that they were lost. Harry refused to accept our situation as such. Luckily for me, I spotted a gas station and said that I needed to get some gas for my trip back into Orange County. Harry accepted my explanation. I was able to have received help from the gas station attendant without embarrassing him. I got Harry to his front door by twelve forty-five.

What happened then really was the shock of the night, not that it was not already filled with enough excitement for one evening....Harry leaned over and tried to kiss me. It was not supposed to be a kiss on the cheek, but out of instinct I had turned my face, and that made him quite mad. He began to spout out some words that were best described as vulgar and most un-gentlemanly. I had a long fuse when it came to my own temper, but when I lost it, watch out!! I slapped Harry so hard that his teeth rattled. Good thing he must have used a good dental adhesive, or they would have gone flying out of his mouth. Harry got out of my car. And I speed away without looking back.

I decided to skip the last game of my season's ticket. Anyway, I had had enough three strikes and you're out ….

Story Twenty-four: Hello It's Me

When I have lived in a large town or city for several years, I was bound to run across people that I had not seen in a long time. Because of my poor memory, I would have found myself feeling embarrassed when the person standing in front of me seemed to remember everything, like we were best buddies. While I stood there racking my brain, as I tried to put a name to their face. Added to my embarrassment, if it was a man, would be the probability that I had actually been out on a date with him and possibly even kissed him goodnight.

Such was the case with Artie and me. Almost every Sunday morning I headed down to Costa Mesa. There was one of the largest outdoor swap meets at the Orange County Fairgrounds. Even if I had nothing to buy, I loved to walk the entire swap meet and browsed. I had just turned down an isle, when a man came up to me with a big smile and friendly greeting:"Well hi, Shelley it's so good to see you". All I did was returned his smile and said something unimportant, while I desperately attempted to recall who he was. If only it was acceptable to say, "Excuse me, but how did I know you?" right then and there. I simply could not have gotten those words out. Instead, I nodded and said "I'm fine, and how were you?"

We were actually walking in opposite directions, when he spotted me in the crowd of browsers and shoppers. If I had been luckier, he would have continued on and I would have been able to go on my way. Wondering all the while "who was that man"?. On that particular Sunday, I was not so fortunate. Artie decided to change course and walked along side of me. I tried to get interested in something hanging on one of the stalls, while I tried to think of a clever way to ask how he knew me. Hoping that the question would not have seemed too rude, I was just about to ask how long had it been since we had last seen each other. When out of his mouth came: "How was my twin's screen play coming along?" Now that simple sentence revealed quite a lot to me. First that he knew that I had a twin, and about a very important project that she had worked on. I wouldn't have walked up to just anyone I met and said "Hi, my name was Shelley and I have an identical twin." Ironically, my sister thought I should have done exactly that. Immediately I began to do some mental replays to see if I could have pictured myself telling the story about my sister to anyone that resembled him. As hard as I tried, my mind was a total blank.

I must have been taking too long to answer, because his face got a worried expression and said "Was everything OK with her? He thought I that I had looked so perplexed. Boy was I! His concern seemed genuine, and only added to my frustration. How could I have forgotten such a nice man. And how could I have told him so? I could not have continued on without spilling the beans. I took a deep breath and said he seemed to know a lot about me, so I only hoped that he also knew that I had an awful memory. I was truly sorry that I could not have recalled his name.

Then I stood still and hoped that he would be understanding and let me off the hook. He looked deep into my eyes for such a long time, I thought I would break into hives with the surge of histamine that was running through my blood. Then he spoke in a very small, almost child-like voice, "You really don't remember me?" Slowly and sadly I nodded my head. I could not have looked back into his rejected face, I started to play with a stone on the ground just to keep me from crying. I felt terrible. But as bad as I thought I was feeling, it only worsened with his next sentence. "Shelley you were so helpful to me and my family when my mother died four years ago, I could never have forgotten you or your kindness." Just as he was about to have said another word… "ARTIE" came to mind. Praise the Lord, I felt as if a weight had finally been lifted. I was so absorbed with my own thoughts, I did not here what he had said…..I had cooked meals for his brothers, and had helped pack up his mom's place after the funeral.

My posture changed immediately. I was able to return his eye contact. I was certain that my facial expression softened too. "How was Jordan doing?" I asked softly. Then I added he was just five at that time, and I remembered it was hardest on him. Artie then knew that my memory had returned. We hugged and continued to walk through the swap stalls, as we talked and laughed. After three hours, I had to leave. We exchanged business cards with our personal numbers written on the back. We both said that we would call soon and keep in touch……

Story Twenty-five: JJ and Henrietta

JJ was a toy frog and he was a very special pet. Stuffed with beans on the inside and soft green flannel as an outer casing, it was a cute looking animal. His eyes were fluffy balls of cotton. As dolls go, JJ had a remarkable quality to be able to make people feel better. My older sister Jackie had convinced me that JJ had special powers, similar to that of the children's tale of the prince that was turned into a frog. She had me believing that if I kept JJ with me all the time, that good things would have happened. And so I did. I went through high school with JJ balanced over my shoulder. As the years went on JJ's insides had gotten worn and frazzled. When it came time to dissect frogs, one of the school pranksters stole JJ and cut him open. It was a sad day for me. The home economics teacher took sympathy on me and had her class patch JJ back together. After her class, JJ had looked better than before the dissection. The students had refilled him with fresh beans and replaced his tired eyes with brand new ones. Indirectly the prankster had done JJ a favor.

JJ became somewhat of an icon. In each class, the students would address JJ as if he had really existed. Everyone wanted to have JJ perched on their shoulders during exams. I was a straight A student and I told everyone that JJ was my lucky charm. It seemed cooler to say that, than having to admit to the long tedious hours I slaved over my studies.

During my high school graduation, I had even gotten the principal to shake JJ's tiny arm when I went up to get my diploma. While filming the ceremony my father got it all on tape, and he was not impressed with my shenanigans.

In my yearbook, I could have been known as the egghead, or as one-half of an identical twin pair, but most of the kids knew me as the proud owner of JJ the frog. Being from Baltimore, being a twin was not a big deal. In fact with a graduating class of 675 students, we had many *sets* of twins and three sets of triplets. There were rumors that something in the water had caused it…no one really knew for sure, but that was a lot of multiple births for one tiny school in one small city. I much preferred the recognition of being known as JJ's owner.

Twenty years had gone by and I lived 3,000 miles across the country. In all that time I had not run into anyone from my school. That situation was about to change. Early one morning I ran out of my favorite perfume, *Shalimar*. After I closed my salon I decided to go shopping at the Brea mall to pick up a few items and restock my cabinets with all of my Shalimar products. All of the major department stores carried it, so I went into Nordstroms. As I walked up to the cosmetic counter, I was greeted by a young woman with the most creatively painted face. Being a make-up artist myself, I quickly noticed the details in the design of her overly dramatic presentation. The clerk had taken stage make-up to an all time high level. I was very surprised that a department store would have tolerated such a harsh appearance of one of it's employees. Since I

had worked in other cosmetic counters, I was aware of the strict guidelines that were normally required.

It was impossible *not* to stare. In trying to cover up for my obvious
reaction, I said to her: "My you certainly have put a lot of time into your
creative make-up expression." She gave me a big toothy grin and her top
three teeth were all capped in gold. That only added to her dramatic
look. What she said next took me by complete surprise. "Didn't you go
to Woodlawn?" That was the name of my high school. I had an awful
memory and did not think I could have recognized any student from
twenty years ago. Even if they were not all made up as she had been, I
don't think I would have recognized anyone. She had a name badge on
and it read "Henrietta". There was no way that I was going to be able to
figure out how I knew her. I decided to be direct and simply admitted
that I did not remember. "I could not believe what an awesome memory
you must have, since it was so very long ago." I said sheepishly. Certainly
we both had changed a good deal since then. I said: "Please forgive me
Henrietta, which of my classes were you in?" She laughed a deep throaty
laugh. It sounded strange coming out of her. My face must have
registered my reaction and my puzzlement. Henrietta blurted out; "You
were the one with the stuffed frog over your shoulder. You dragged it
everywhere. JJ was it's name, right?" I nodded affirmatively. Then she
continued on, by saying that I had a lot of people convinced that JJ
made me smart. Although she had never bought that line of crap.
Henrietta went on reliving our past history as she said "I remembered
seeing you come into the library when it opened and not leaving until it
closed." I still could not place her at all. Then she dropped the other
bomb-shell. "You mentioned a moment ago that we must have all
changed a lot since high school, I knew that I certainly had. Back then
you would have called me Hank. I had gone through the complete sex
change years ago, and I'm now legally Henrietta." She let the last
sentence have it's full impact on me and stared so hard, her eyes felt like

they were burning holes through my cheeks. My face flushed with embarrassment and confusion. I did not know what to say. Maybe that was why her make-up did not seem out of place to her. Perhaps through all the changes she was forced to go through, wearing outlandish make-up seemed mild and conservative. I felt odd, so I purchased all of my products and quickly left the store. If nothing else came of our brief encounter, Henrietta would have enjoyed the fat commission she earned through my sale. Since I was so uncomfortable, and not knowing what I should have said or done, I found myself buying three times the volume of bottles than what I had planned. I left Nordstroms with two full shopping bags of every product in the Shalimar line and a credit card bill over three hundred dollars.

Perhaps something's in our past are best to stay in our past....

Synopsis of Sex Lust and No Fat—
A personal journey in the 90's

Chapter One: First Dates

The four stories told of unique and funny encounters. Story Three described how a long term relationship enfolded from a bizarre twist of fate.

Chapter Two: Romance and Dancing

These four stories presented the splendor that dancing offered, even with strangers. Some helpful hints were shared to handle "mashers" and "overzealous partners" while on the dance floor.

Chapter Three: Creative Ways To Meet Mr. Right?

Nine humorous stories covered the gambit of ways to seek out great dates. All women would laugh and cry over the situations that happened during my search for the perfect partner.

Chapter Four: Dining and Dieting

These two stories depicted the perils that faced all women that need to lose weight while dating. Clever alternatives were given to help women diet and still have an active social life.

Chapter Five: Unique Experiences For a Single Woman

Being single offered opportunities for adventure. These six stories shared some of my best situations while vacationing, during the holidays and other unique events.